SUPER CLEAN SUPER FOODS

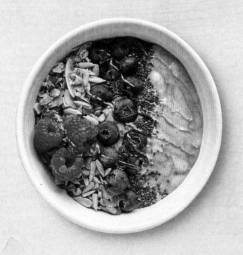

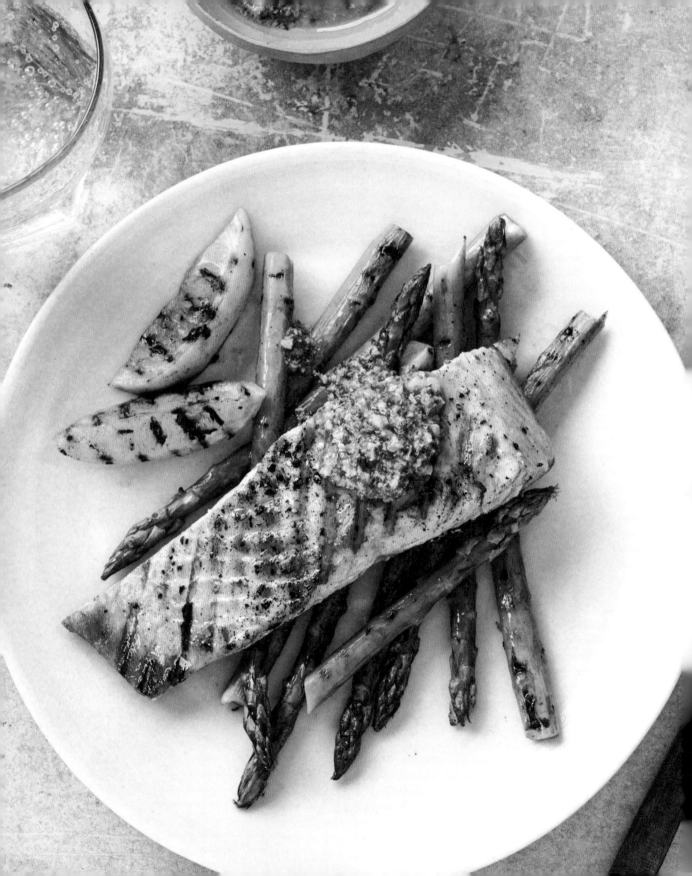

SUPER CLEAN SUPER FOODS

FIONA HUNTER
CAROLINE BRETHERTON

CONTENTS

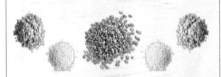

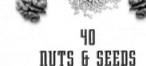
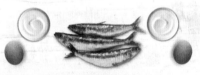

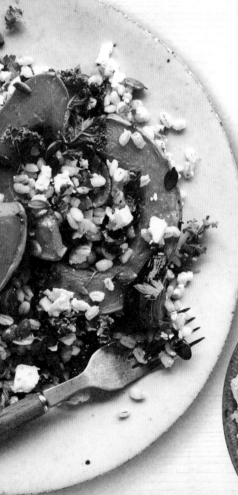
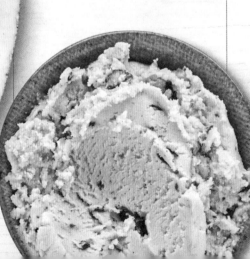

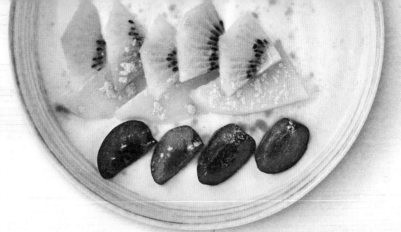

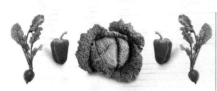

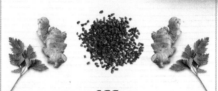

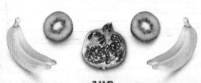

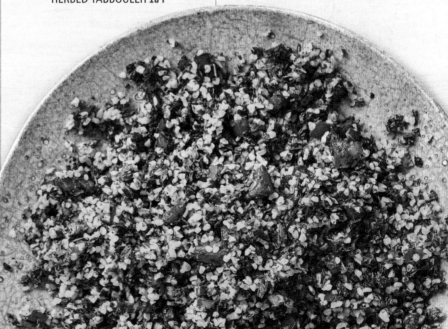

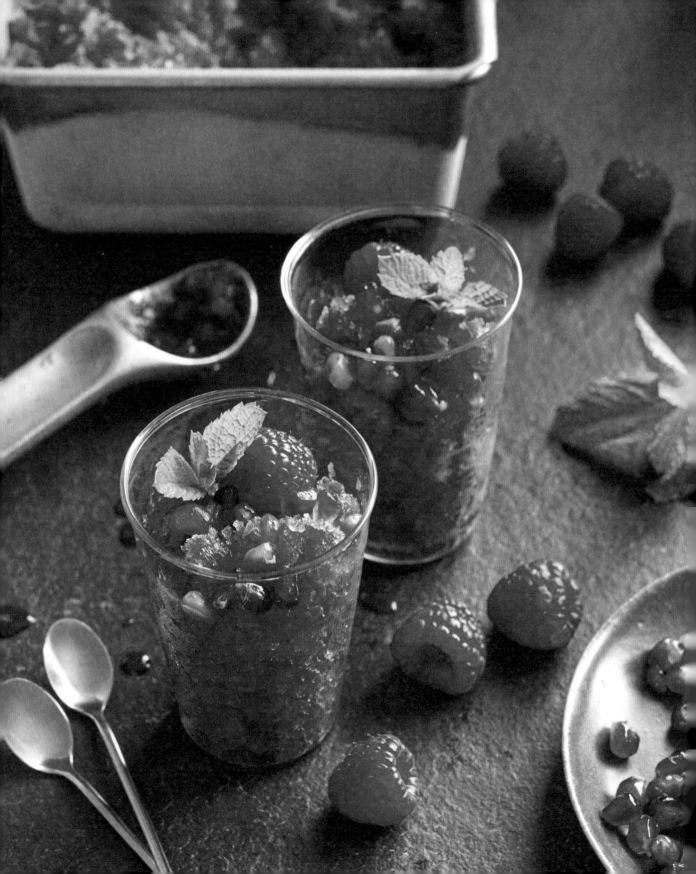

FOREWORD

Super-Clean Superfoods is your guide to the world's healthiest foods.
It'll show you how to pack your diet with superfoods in the healthiest and
most delicious way possible. The foods you eat have a fundamental impact
on your health and well-being, both in the short and long term. Eating
a healthy, balanced diet is a vital investment that will improve
your chances of living a long and healthy life.

This book is a visual directory of 90 of the most important superfoods—
foods so nutrient-dense that they warrant the term. Each superfood in
this book comes with information on which key nutrients it contains and
how they benefit your body, as well as simple, delicious ideas for how to
incorporate it into your diet and tips for maximizing its nutritional benefits.

Too often, superfoods come with an aura of mystique that makes them
seem inaccessible, expensive, or difficult to cook. Simple ingredients, such
as carrots, beets, almonds, and chicken, are tasty, easily accessible, and
packed with health-boosting vitamins, minerals, and phytochemicals.
For more adventurous eaters, we have also included harder-to-find
superfoods, such as dulse flakes, acai powder, and spirulina.

Interspersed throughout the book are 20 superfood-packed recipes,
as well as ideas for how to eat for a healthy gut, good sleep, brain power,
immunity boost, glowing skin, and extra energy.

We hope this book demystifies superfoods and clean eating, and helps
you eat more nutritious, tasty foods every day.

FIONA HUNTER   **CAROLINE BRETHERTON**

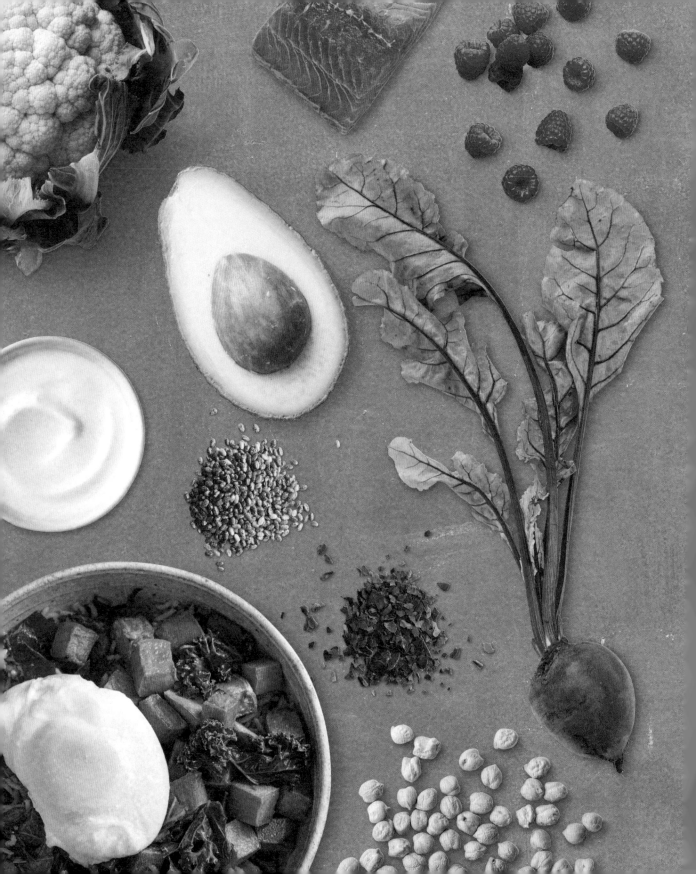

SUPER-CLEAN EATING

WHAT IS A SUPERFOOD?

There are foods that are so packed with nutrients that they deserve to be called "super," and you're missing out if you don't include them in your diet. These foods are packed with health-boosting vitamins, minerals, and phytochemicals.

WHAT MAKES A FOOD "SUPER"?

The food you eat provides your body with the fuel it needs for energy, the building blocks for growth and repair of tissues, and tools that protect cells and organs from disease. Superfoods are simply foods that deliver impressive quantities of these health-promoting nutrients.

They are foods that are packed with **vitamins**, **minerals**, **antioxidants**, **phytochemicals**, **fiber**, or **healthy fats**.

They are foods that are known to help protect against a whole host of diseases, and that help make your heart healthier, your brain sharper, and your immune system stronger. They can improve your well-being and help you stay active and healthy as you grow older. They are a group of foods that you must have in your diet if you want to improve your chances of living a long and healthy life.

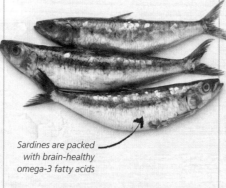

Sardines are packed with brain-healthy omega-3 fatty acids

HOW DO I CHOOSE WHICH TO EAT?

The good news is that superfoods don't have to be new and exotic, hard to find, or expensive in order to be beneficial.

Carrots are just as much of a **superfood** as more exotic ingredients like **spirulina** or **acai powder**.

There are plenty of superfoods to choose from, so if you don't like the taste of a particular food or your budget doesn't stretch to some of the more expensive ingredients, this book will help you discover other superfoods that offer similar nutrients and benefits.

HOW OFTEN SHOULD I EAT THEM?

Whatever your **age** or **circumstances**, you should strive to **include** some **superfoods** in your **diet every day**.

It's never too early or too late to start incorporating superfoods into your diet. Some of the superfoods set you up for lifelong good health, and others may even help reverse existing cell damage. Try to incorporate 3–4 superfoods into your meals every day, and vary them from week to week. No single superfood contains all the nutrients you need, so eat a variety of superfoods rather than sticking to the same ones.

Phytochemicals in lemons can help improve blood flow to your brain

Avocados contain vitamins that protect your heart

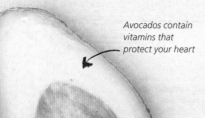

Ginger may help reduce the risk of heart disease

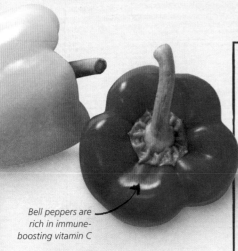

Bell peppers are rich in immune-boosting vitamin C

WILL EATING THEM MAKE ME HEALTHY?

Superfoods are not magic bullets—throwing a few superfoods into a diet that is unhealthy or unbalanced (see pp14–15) won't magically transform your health and well-being.

A **healthy diet** is just one piece of the **puzzle** that makes up a **healthy lifestyle.**

As well as eating clean and supercharging your diet with superfoods, you also need to exercise regularly, keep your weight within the healthy range, drink only moderate quantities of alcohol (if you drink at all), and don't smoke.

Superfoods are more beneficial than nutrition supplements. Eating fresh, organic foods provides a whole host of nutrients that you wouldn't get from swallowing a pill—even if food does take a little longer to prepare. Most superfoods contain a cocktail of active ingredients, and it is the interaction between these ingredients that offers the health benefits.

Incorporating the **superfoods** into your diet is **simple,** as well as being much more **delicious** than taking vitamin **supplements**.

SUPERFOOD BENEFITS

Different superfoods provide distinct benefits for your body. These icons provide an at-a-glance guide to the key health benefits of each superfood.

 GOOD SLEEP
Superfoods rich in magnesium, calcium, or tryptophan help your body manufacture sleep hormones, helping you get a good night's sleep.

 BRAIN POWER
Phytochemicals found in superfoods help improve blood flow to your brain. Omega-3 fatty acids also help keep your brain healthy.

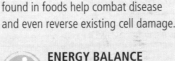 **DISEASE PREVENTION**
Numerous phytochemicals, antioxidants, and selenium found in foods help combat disease and even reverse existing cell damage.

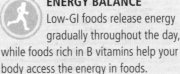 **ENERGY BALANCE**
Low-GI foods release energy gradually throughout the day, while foods rich in B vitamins help your body access the energy in foods.

 BLOOD HEALTH
Foods packed with folate, iron, vitamin K, or nitrates help your body produce and maintain healthy blood.

 HEART HEALTH
Healthy fats and phytochemicals, as well as whole grains, help reduce the risk of heart disease and stroke.

 DIGESTIVE HEALTH
Different types of fiber help keep your digestive system healthy, while fermented foods encourage gut-friendly bacteria.

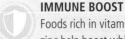 **IMMUNE BOOST**
Foods rich in vitamin C or zinc help boost white blood cells that combat disease and infection.

 HORMONE BALANCE
Iodine-rich foods help your body regulate hormones. Some superfoods contain phytochemicals that can alleviate menopausal symptoms.

 BONE, JOINT, AND MUSCLE STRENGTH
Superfoods that are packed with calcium, vitamin K, and magnesium support your skeleton and muscles.

 EYE HEALTH
Vitamin A and phytochemicals called carotenoids help protect your eyes against free-radical damage and cataracts.

ANTI-AGING
Beta-carotene in foods protects your skin against signs of aging, and protein-rich foods help protect against muscle wastage.

 SKIN HEALTH
Superfoods rich in vitamins E, A, and C, as well as beta-carotene, support your skin.

HOW TO EAT CLEAN

Clean eating is simple: it means eating foods that are unprocessed or minimally processed. There's no need to eat only raw foods, or cut particular food groups out of your diet—just embrace the whole range of superfoods available.

CLEAN THINKING

Clean eating requires a little forethought. Plan your meals for the week, and make sure that your shopping bags are filled with fresh fruit and vegetables, healthy proteins, and whole grains. Avoid most processed foods, as these usually contain added salt, sugar, or fat, and lower levels of nutrients.

For many **people**, choosing to **"eat clean"** involves a **change** of **mindset**.

It's easy to be put off clean eating because it seems less convenient than a store-bought meal or takeout. A clean diet does take a little more effort than speedy eating, but if you want to look after your body and improve your chances of living a long and healthy life, you need to spend time and energy getting your diet right.

MAKE POSITIVE CHANGES

Once you get the hang of it, you'll discover that clean eating doesn't have to be time-consuming, expensive, complicated, or restrictive, and it doesn't mean shunning all convenience foods.

Some **processed foods**, such as canned **tomatoes** and canned **fish**, are highly nutritious and are not heavily **processed** or stuffed with **additives**.

Take time to think about the ingredients you use, check ingredient lists, and see if you can find more wholesome, nutritious versions of your food essentials.

Clean eating isn't about trading pleasure for health. You don't have to be squeaky-clean and virtuous all the time—it's what you eat most of the time that's important. A clean diet allows you to enjoy the true flavors of food, and choose foods that are better for your body and for the environment.

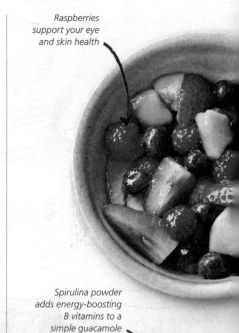

Raspberries support your eye and skin health

Spirulina powder adds energy-boosting B vitamins to a simple guacamole

Shiitake mushrooms contain a unique phytochemical that helps lower cholesterol levels

6 WAYS TO CLEAN UP YOUR DIET

Making a few simple changes to your shopping, cooking, and eating habits can transform your diet. Start with these six steps, and you'll be eating cleaner and feeling healthier in no time.

1 PLAN AHEAD

Invest some time in planning what you are going to eat for the week ahead. This makes it easier to decide what to eat at the end of a long and busy day, and can help you avoid turning to convenience foods.

2 CHECK THE LABEL

If you do buy food in jars or packages, take some time to look at the ingredients list. If you don't recognize anything, or if the list contains more than three ingredients, then put it back on the shelf.

3 FREEZE YOUR OWN PREMADE MEALS

Scale up freezable recipes for things like tomato sauce or vegetable soup. Make double the quantity and freeze half of it for another day.

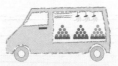

4 EAT SEASONALLY

Food that has had to travel thousands of miles before arriving in your kitchen has usually been selected for its ability to travel rather than its flavor, and has been losing nutrients since the moment it was picked. Seasonal foods usually taste better, and are likely to have travelled less distance to get to you.

5 BUY LOCAL

Shop at your local farmers' market or grocer to find the best foods available in your area. You can also shop online, where you're less likely to be tempted to buy unhealthy food, or shop the the perimeter of the supermarket—most unprocessed, natural foods are on the outside aisles.

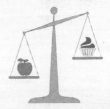

6 EAT 80% CLEAN

It can be difficult to eat clean 100 percent of the time. Try to eat healthily most of the time, in order to give your body the nutrients it needs without feeling deprived.

A BALANCED DIET

Keeping active and eating a superfood-packed, balanced diet maximizes your chances of having a healthy body and living a long life. Build a varied diet from wholesome, nutritious foods from each of these five key groups.

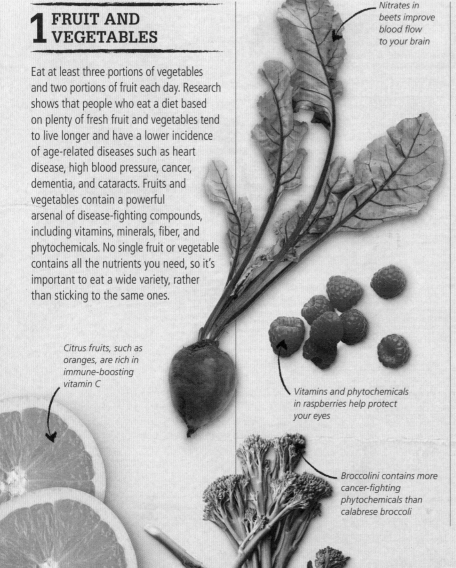

1 FRUIT AND VEGETABLES

Eat at least three portions of vegetables and two portions of fruit each day. Research shows that people who eat a diet based on plenty of fresh fruit and vegetables tend to live longer and have a lower incidence of age-related diseases such as heart disease, high blood pressure, cancer, dementia, and cataracts. Fruits and vegetables contain a powerful arsenal of disease-fighting compounds, including vitamins, minerals, fiber, and phytochemicals. No single fruit or vegetable contains all the nutrients you need, so it's important to eat a wide variety, rather than sticking to the same ones.

Nitrates in beets improve blood flow to your brain

Citrus fruits, such as oranges, are rich in immune-boosting vitamin C

Vitamins and phytochemicals in raspberries help protect your eyes

Broccolini contains more cancer-fighting phytochemicals than calabrese broccoli

2 STARCHY CARBOHYDRATES

Starchy carbohydrates come in different guises and many of the carbohydrates we choose have been stripped of most of their fiber and other nutrients. Refining wheat to produce white flour, for instance, removes more than half of the B vitamins, 90 percent of the vitamin E, and almost all of the fiber. Choose unrefined carbohydrates, such whole grains, beans, and pulses. Aim to eat three portions of unrefined starchy carbohydrates each day.

A type of fiber called beta-glucan, which is found in barley, helps reduce bad cholesterol

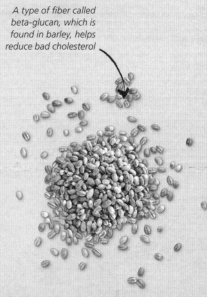

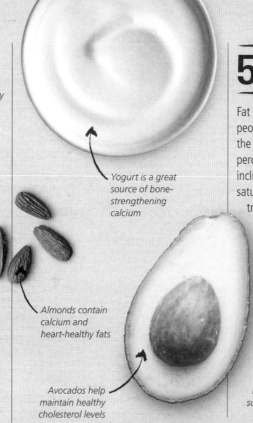

Sesame seeds are a useful source of calcium for people who don't eat dairy

Yogurt is a great source of bone-strengthening calcium

3 CALCIUM-RICH FOODS

Calcium is essential for building strong bones and teeth, and is particularly important while bones are still growing. Aim for at least two portions of calcium each day. Milk and dairy products are a good source of calcium, as well as providing other nutrients such as vitamins A and B2. If you don't eat dairy products, you can get calcium from almonds, fortified soy or nut milk, sesame seeds, kale, broccoli, and bok choy.

Almonds contain calcium and heart-healthy fats

Avocados help maintain healthy cholesterol levels

5 HEALTHY FATS

Fat is essential for your health, but most people consume far too much of it, and the wrong sort. Eat no more than 30 percent of your calories each day from fat, including no more than 11 percent from saturated fat. Avoid saturated fats and trans fats, as these increase levels of bad cholesterol in your blood. Instead, choose unsaturated fats, such as olive and canola oil, and foods such as avocados, nuts, seeds, and oily fish.

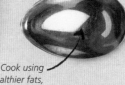

Cook using healthier fats, such as olive or canola oil

4 HEALTHY PROTEINS

Protein should provide 15–20 percent of your total calorie intake each day. Protein is essential for cell growth and repair throughout your life. Choose healthier proteins, such as oily fish, beans, pulses, nuts, and seeds—in addition to protein, these contain other health-promoting nutrients, such as omega-3 fatty acids, vitamins, and minerals.

Black beans are packed with protein and gut-healthy fiber

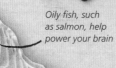

Oily fish, such as salmon, help power your brain

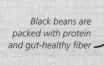

NUTRITIONAL GUIDELINES

Nutritional graphics pick out the key nutrients in the food

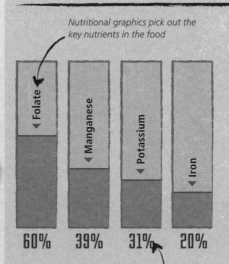

Folate | Manganese | Potassium | Iron

60%   **39%**   **31%**   **20%**

Labels tell you the RI percentage for each nutrient

For each of the superfoods in this book, you'll find a nutritional information chart (see left) featuring the key nutrients found in the superfood. These are nutrients that have a reference intake (RI) based on national guidelines. RIs act as a rough guide to how much of each nutrient you should aim to consume each day. RIs vary based on age, gender, and individual dietary needs (see pp212–13)—percentages in this book are based on RIs for for women aged 19–50. Use these graphics to make sure you get an approximate balance of the key nutrients. Not all nutrients have a specified RI, including phytochemicals, so always read the "Why eat it?" text to give you an overview of the benefits of each superfood.

THE KEY NUTRIENTS

Throughout this book, you'll find reference to these vitamins and minerals, all of which are vital for maintaining a healthy body. Here is a quick guide to the key benefits and sources of each nutrient.

VITAMINS

VITAMIN A (RETINOL)

Needed for: growth and development, and healthy skin, eyes, and immune system.

Key sources: carrots, sweet potato

VITAMIN B1 (THIAMINE)

Needed for: a healthy nervous system and accessing energy in foods.

Key sources: nutritional yeast, barley, oats

VITAMIN B2 (RIBOFLAVIN)

Needed for: accessing energy in foods. May help protect against cataracts.

Key sources: goji berries, mint, cayenne pepper

VITAMIN B3 (NIACIN)

Needed for: a healthy nervous system, and accessing energy in foods. May help improve circulation.

Key sources: chicken, peanuts, fava beans

VITAMIN B5 (PANTHOTHENIC ACID)

Needed for: accessing energy in foods.

Key sources: yogurt, cauliflower, avocado

VITAMIN B6 (PYRIDOXINE)

Needed for: a healthy nervous system and for producing red blood cells. May also help reduce symptoms associated with premenstrual syndrome (PMS).

Key sources: wheat germ, pistachios, avocado, banana, nutritional yeast

VITAMIN B12

Needed for: a healthy nervous system and for producing red blood cells. May also contribute to improving the quality of your sleep.

Key sources: salmon, eggs, nutritional yeast

FOLATE (FOLIC ACID)

Needed for: producing red blood cells, and accessing energy in foods. Protects against neural tube defects in early pregnancy. May also offer protection against breast and colon cancers.

Key sources: asparagus, beets, cabbage, fennel, quinoa

BIOTIN

Needed for: accessing energy in foods. May also keep your nails and hair healthy.

Key sources: almonds

VITAMIN C (ASCORBIC ACID)

Needed for: protecting the cells that make up your immune system and boosting the action of bacteria- and virus-combating white blood cells. Supports your skin and eye health. May also protect against cancer, heart disease, and stroke.

Key sources: red bell peppers, broccoli, strawberries, oranges, lemons

VITAMIN D (CHOLECALCIFEROL)

Needed for: healthy nervous, immune, and skeletal systems. May reduce the risk of osteoporosis and bone fracture.

Key sources: salmon, eggs

VITAMIN E (TOCOPHEROLS)

Needed for: healthy eyes, skin, heart, and immune system. May help protect against prostate cancer and cataracts.

Key sources: sunflower seeds, almonds, avocado, pine nuts

VITAMIN K

Needed for: strong bones and healthy blood. May help protect against osteoporosis, osteoarthritis, stroke, and heart disease.

Key sources: cabbage, broccoli, cilantro, parsley, asparagus

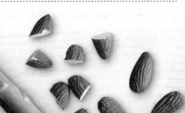

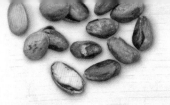

MINERALS

CALCIUM

Needed for: blood clotting and strong bones and teeth. May help prevent high blood pressure and protect against prostate and colon cancers.

Key sources: yogurt, sesame seeds, almonds, figs

CHROMIUM

Needed for: regulating blood sugar levels and keeping your heart healthy. May help improve insulin resistance and glucose control for people with diabetes.

Key sources: pistachios

COPPER

Needed for: healthy bones, blood, and nervous system. May help prevent high cholesterol.

Key sources: buckwheat, shiitake mushrooms, goji berries, cashews

MAGNESIUM

Needed for: healthy bones, accessing energy in foods, and nerve and muscle function. Helps protect against heart disease, stroke, and high blood pressure. May also help prevent diabetes.

Key sources: barley, buckwheat, mustard seeds, cacao nibs

PHOSPHORUS

Needed for: healthy bones and teeth and accessing energy in foods.

Key sources: amaranth, brown rice, garlic, cashews, coconut

POTASSIUM

Needed for: the transmission of nerve impulses and keeping your heart beating. Helps maintain healthy blood pressure. May help reduce the risk of stroke and osteoporosis.

Key sources: fennel, sweet potato, avocado, banana

IRON

Needed for: manufacturing hemoglobin, the protein in blood that carries oxygen around your body. Iron may help increase energy levels.

Key sources: teff, kale, amaranth, goji berries, moringa powder, turmeric

ZINC

Needed for: growth, reproduction, wound healing, and a healthy immune system. May help protect against age-related macular degeneration, which is the most common cause of loss of eyesight in older people.

Key sources: chlorella, pumpkin seeds, oats, thyme

MANGANESE

Needed for: many of the chemical processes that occur in your body, including energy production. May help control blood sugar levels and prevent osteoporosis.

Key sources: buckwheat, amaranth, pine nuts, brown rice

IODINE

Needed for: manufacturing thyroid hormones, which are needed for growth and regulating your metabolism.

Key sources: wakame, nori, eggs

SELENIUM

Needed for: a healthy immune system. May help reduce the risk of cancer, lower high cholesterol levels, and protect against heart disease and arthritis.

Key sources: Brazil nuts, barley, salmon, eggs

PHYTOCHEMICALS

Phytochemicals are naturally occurring chemicals found in foods of plant origin. Many of the special health benefits of the superfoods come from these nutrients. There are hundreds of phytochemicals—here are some of the most well-known:

• **Carotenoids** such as beta-carotene, lycopene, lutein, and zeaxanthin are found in fruit and vegetables with orange, red, and yellow flesh. They help keep your skin, eyes, and heart healthy.

• **Polyphenols**, such as catechins, may help prevent cell damage.

• **Bioflavonoids** are powerful antioxidants found in citrus fruits that help your body absorb vitamin C.

• **Flavonoids**, which include anthocyanins and flavonols such as rutin and quercetin, help reduce high blood pressure, improve blood flow to your brain, and may reduce the risk of some types of cancer.

• **Phytosterols** help reduce levels of bad cholesterol in your blood.

• **Phytoestrogens**, including lignans and coumestans, may help protect against cancer and reduce symptoms associated with menopause.

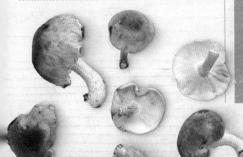

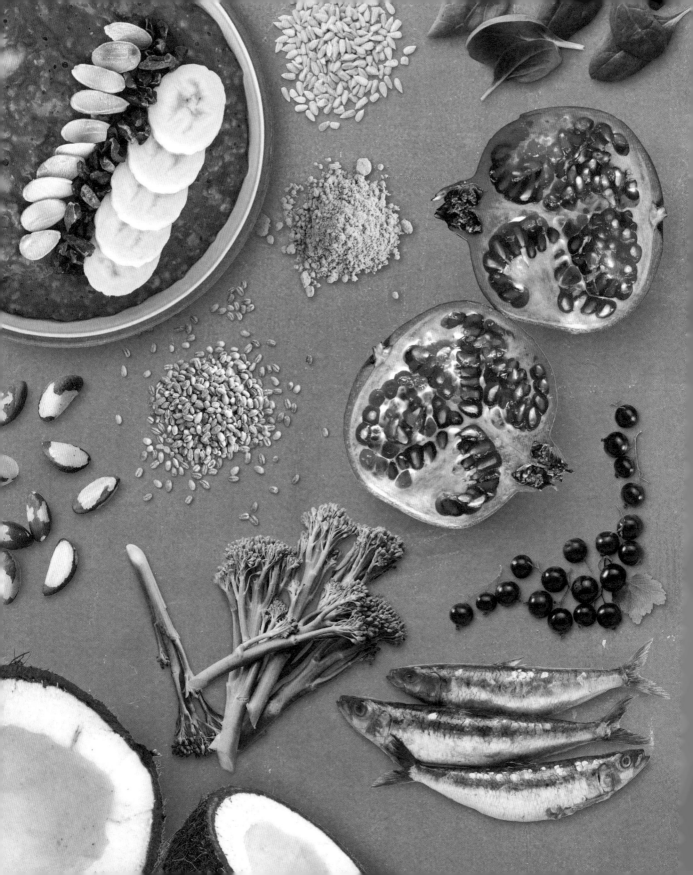

THE
SUPERFOODS

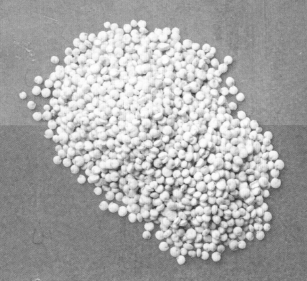

GRAINS

OATS

Providing more soluble fiber than any other grain, oats also contain slow-release, low-GI carbohydrates. Oats are also rich in beta-glucan, which helps reduce high cholesterol and maintain blood sugar levels, and vitamin B1, which helps your body convert food into energy.

WHY EAT IT?

HEART HEALTH
Beta-glucan is a form of fiber that dissolves in your digestive tract, forming a gel that binds to excess cholesterol and prevents it from being absorbed into the blood. Studies show that eating ½ teaspoon (3g) of beta-glucan per day for just 4 weeks can reduce high cholesterol levels by up to 10 percent.

CANCER PREVENTION
Studies show that people who eat three or more servings of whole grains, such as oats, per day have a reduced risk of certain types of cancer, heart disease, and type 2 diabetes.

ENERGY BALANCE
Beta-glucan is a type of fiber that helps to slow the absorption of sugar into the blood—this means that oats give a sustained release of sugar. This helps to prevent spikes in blood sugar levels and slowly releases energy for your body throughout the day. Beta-glucan and magnesium can also help to regulate insulin secretion—a benefit for those with diabetes.

The **beta-glucan** in oats prevents **cholesterol** from being absorbed into your **blood**, and may **reduce** high cholesterol by **up to 10 percent**.

WHAT'S IN IT?

A ½-cup serving of oats is a good source of beta-glucan, vitamin B1, magnesium, and zinc. Oats also contain protein, vitamins B2 and B6, niacin, calcium, folate, potassium, iron, phosphorus, and selenium.

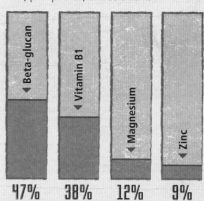

Beta-glucan	Vitamin B1	Magnesium	Zinc
47%	38%	12%	9%

Percentage of your daily reference intake

Whole oats are rich in fiber, which supports good digestive health

TIP
Keep whole grains in an airtight container. Heat, light, and moisture can degrade healthy oils.

WHERE IS IT FROM?

The oat, also called the common oat, is part of the cereal grain family and is grown in temperate regions for its seed. Oat was seen as a weedlike plant for centuries before domesticated oats appeared during the Bronze Age in Europe.

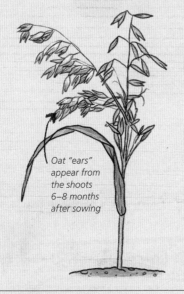

Oat "ears" appear from the shoots 6–8 months after sowing

MAXIMIZE THE BENEFITS

ROLLED OATS
Choose steel-cut oats or traditional rolled oats instead of quick-cook instant oats, which are more heavily processed and often include added sugar.

MAKE YOUR OWN OATMEAL
For a healthy, homemade alternative to processed, "quick-cook" oatmeal, simply blend rolled oats in a food processor until they are partially broken down, then cook as usual.

HOW TO EAT IT

1 OATCAKES
Traditional oatcakes hail from Scotland and are delicious served with hummus or nut butter. Make your own using oatmeal, bound together with a little whole-wheat flour, olive oil, and seasoning.

2 MAKE PANCAKES
Oats make a fantastic alternative to flour in breakfast pancakes. Blend the oats to a fine powder and mix with egg, milk, grated apple, a little honey, and baking powder for delicious apple and oat pancakes.

3 CRANBERRY AND OAT COOKIES
Every once in a while a cookie is a good thing. To enhance the flavor and benefits, add into your mixture a couple of handfuls of superfood nuts and dried fruits, such as pistachios and cranberries.

The high quantities of **beta-glucan** in **oats** help to **slow** the **aborption** of sugar into your **blood**. This **prevents** spikes in **blood sugar**, and helps keep your **energy levels balanced** throughout the day.

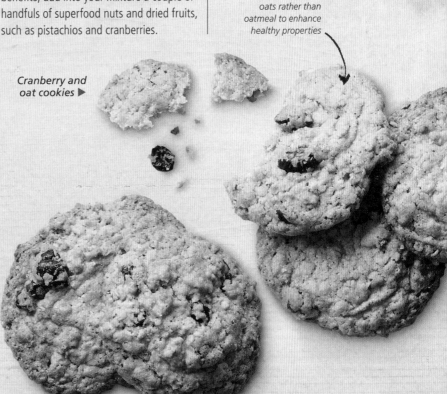

Use whole rolled oats rather than oatmeal to enhance healthy properties

Cranberry and oat cookies ▶

SUPERSEED GRANOLA

This breakfast is based on nourishing oats, which provide slow-release energy and help reduce high levels of cholesterol in the blood. Nuts and seeds provide healthy fats and phytochemicals that benefit your heart.

Makes 7-8 cups, about 12 portions · **Prep time** 15 minutes · **Cook time** 30–35 minutes

INGREDIENTS

2 tbsp coconut oil

⅓ cup maple syrup

¼ tsp fine salt

1 tsp ground **cinnamon**

3½ cups rolled **oats**

½ cup **pumpkin seeds**

¼ cup **sunflower seeds**

¾ cup sliced **almonds**

¾ cup hazelnuts, coarsely chopped

1 cup dried fruit, such as **cranberries**, **cherries**, raisins, and pitted dates, coarsely chopped

½ cup toasted coconut chips

1 tbsp **chia seeds**

1 tbsp golden **flaxseeds**

METHOD

1 Preheat the oven to 325°F (160°C). If the coconut oil is solid, melt it in a small saucepan. Once melted, remove it from the heat and whisk in the maple syrup, salt, and cinnamon.

2 Mix the oats, pumpkin seeds, sunflower seeds, and nuts together in a large bowl. Pour the maple syrup liquid over the dried mixture and toss it very well to combine.

3 Spread the granola mixture over two large baking sheets. Place in the center of the oven and bake for 30–40 minutes, turning every 10 minutes. Ensure that the granola is spread out, so that it browns evenly. The granola is ready when it is golden brown and crunchy.

4 Let the granola cool, then mix in the dried fruit, toasted coconut chips, chia seeds, and flaxseeds. Serve with yogurt or milk and fresh fruit. You can store the granola in an airtight container for up to 2 weeks.

SUPER SWAP

• Exchange chia seeds for energy-boosting amaranth, baking it with the oats

• Use dried pineapple, mango, and papaya for their gut-healthy fiber

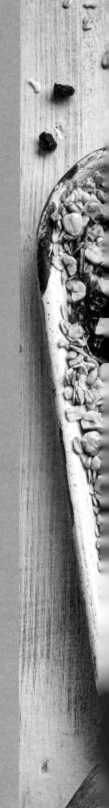

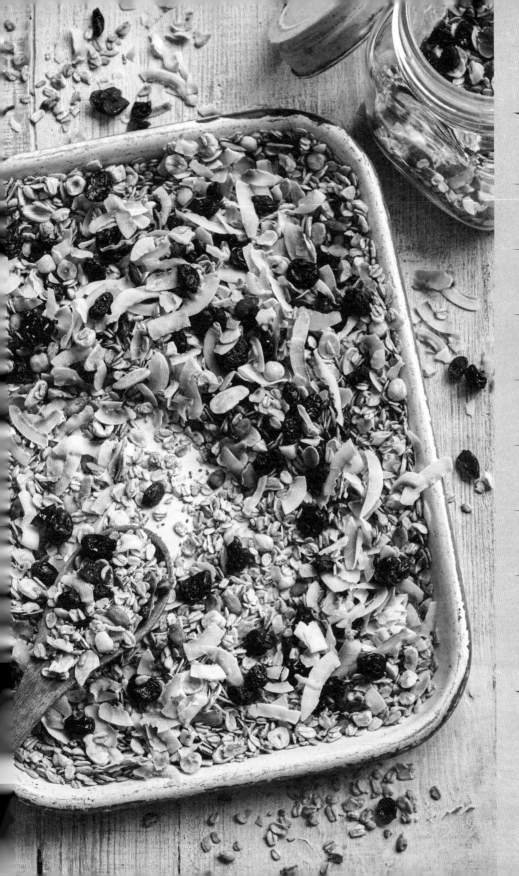

FEATURED SUPERFOODS

CINNAMON
helps **lower blood sugar levels**

OATS
help reduce **high cholesterol**

PUMPKIN SEEDS
are good for **skin health**

SUNFLOWER SEEDS
help increase **good cholesterol**

ALMONDS
reduce the risk of **heart disease**

CRANBERRIES
prevent recurrent **urinary tract infections**

CHIA SEEDS
help keep your **heart healthy**

FLAXSEEDS
help reduce **menopausal symptoms**

Nutrition per serving

Energy 307cals (1234kj)
Carbohydrate 29g
– of which sugars 11g
Fiber 4g
Fat 17g
– of which saturated 5g
Salt 0.1g
Protein 8g
Cholesterol 0g

WHEAT GERM

The wheat grain's germ contains all the fuel that the plant needs to grow—it is a concentrated high-fiber source of manganese and energy-boosting B vitamins.

WHY EAT IT?

HIGH IN MANGANESE
The high levels of manganese in wheat germ support many of the chemical processes that happen in the body, including energy production, helping support blood, brain, and nerve health.

ENERGY BALANCE
Rich in B vitamins, wheat germ helps your body convert energy from food into energy your body can use.

DIGESTIVE HEALTH
Wheat germ is a good source of both soluble fiber, which helps reduce high cholesterol levels and slow the release of sugar into your blood, and insoluble fiber, which helps speed passage of waste material through the digestive tract, helping to prevent constipation.

Wheat germ is the part of the plant that grows into wheatgrass

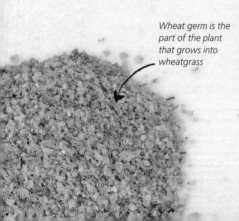

WHAT'S IN IT?

A 2-tablespoon serving of wheat germ is an excellent source of manganese, and a good source of vitamins B6, B1, and E. It also contains vitamin B2, niacin, and folate.

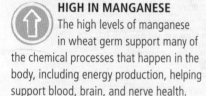

Manganese ▲	Vitamin B6 ▲	Vitamin B1 ▲	Vitamin E ▲
101%	28%	25%	20%

Percentage of your daily reference intake

WHERE IS IT FROM?

The germ is the part of the wheat kernel that grows into a new plant. The rest of the starchy kernel is milled for flour.

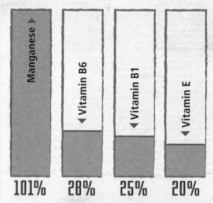

The germ sits inside layers of protein and fiber in the kernel

HOW TO EAT IT

1 ADD TO A SMOOTHIE
Wheat germ has a mild, sweet flavor—put 1 tablespoon of it into your breakfast smoothie for added fiber.

2 BREAKFAST BARS
Raw energy bars make a great snack or on-the-go breakfast. Add extra nutrients to homemade energy bars (see pp48–49) with a handful of wheat germ.

3 IN GRANOLA
Add wheat germ to homemade granola. Mix a handful or two into the granola along with the dried fruit after it comes out of the oven—the wheat germ will burn if baked with the oats and nuts.

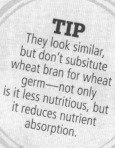

TIP
They look similar, but don't subsitute wheat bran for wheat germ—not only is it less nutritious, but it reduces nutrient absorption.

TEFF

Rich in vitamin B1, iron, and resistant starch, teff supports your nervous system, blood, and digestive tract. It is also gluten-free and high in protein.

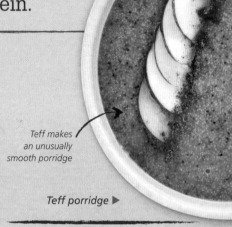

Teff makes an unusually smooth porridge

Teff porridge ▶

WHY EAT IT?

DIGESTIVE HEALTH
Some 20–40 percent of the starch in teff is resistant starch which, passing through the digestive tract undigested, helps keep the colon healthy and encourages the growth of friendly bacteria. Because resistant starch is slowly fermented, it is better tolerated and produces less flatulence than some other types of fiber.

HORMONE BALANCE
Teff has a low glycemic index (GI), which means that your body converts it into sugar more slowly than many other carbohydrates—it gradually releases sugar into your blood, providing long-lasting energy for your body. This makes teff a good choice for people with diabetes.

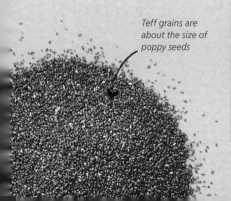

Teff grains are about the size of poppy seeds

WHAT'S IN IT?

A ¾-cup serving of cooked teff is a good source of vitamin B1, iron, fiber, and potassium. It also contains vitamins B2 and B6, as well as protein.

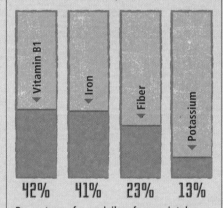

Vitamin B1 — Iron — Fiber — Potassium

42%   41%   23%   13%

Percentage of your daily reference intake

WHERE IS IT FROM?

Teff is the seed of a grass native to Ethiopia. In Ethiopia it is ground to a flour and fermented to make injera, a thin, spongy, sourdough flatbread.

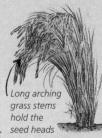

Long arching grass stems hold the seed heads

HOW TO EAT IT

1 TEFF PORRIDGE
Use teff in place of oats for a fiber-rich porridge. Bring teff grains to a boil in water, then simmer for 10 minutes. Stir in a little almond milk, ground cinnamon, and honey, and top with slices of apple.

2 IN PLACE OF POLENTA
The smooth texture of teff makes it an ideal substitute for polenta. Cook it with vegetable stock and plenty of seasoning, as you would polenta.

3 VEGAN BURGERS
Combine cooked teff grain with chopped herbs and scallions, then form into patties and let cool. Bake in the oven and serve in whole-wheat bread buns with salad leaves, sliced tomato, and your choice of sauces.

EATING FOR GUT HEALTH

Imbalances in gut flora are thought to be at the root of many chronic diseases. A healthy gut is the foundation of a healthy body—so it makes sense to look after your digestive health. Here is an example of a day of eating for gut health, incorporating foods that boost your digestion into every meal.

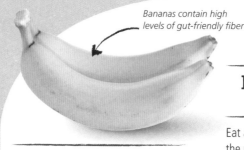

Bananas contain high levels of gut-friendly fiber

TO DRINK

Making sure your body is well hydrated will help keep your gut healthy by preventing constipation. The insoluble fiber found in vegetables and whole grains—vital for a healthy digestive tract—only works efficiently when it has absorbed water. Add fresh mint to hot or cold water to ease an upset stomach or bloating.

Water infused with mint helps soothe your stomach

BREAKFAST

Breakfast provides the perfect opportunity to stock up on one very important group of gut-friendly superfoods: whole grains. Whole grains, such as oats and wheatgerm, provide insoluble fiber, which speeds up the passage of waste material and toxins through your digestive tract.

Fiber-rich, whole-grain cereals support your digestive health

MID-MORNING SNACK

Eat a banana halfway through the morning to boost your digestive health. Bananas contain a particularly helpful type of prebiotic fiber called fructooligosaccharides (FOS). FOS nourish and encourage the growth of good bacteria in the gut, helping them to crowd out the bad bacteria that cause digestive problems.

Layer fruit with yogurt to make a healthy snack

AFTERNOON SNACK

The bacteria in probiotic yogurt and fermented dairy products such as kefir boost levels of good bacteria in the gut, so eat as a snack with fiber-rich fruit. Good bacteria break down fiber into short-chain fatty acids, which help protect against inflammation.

Eat fermented
Fermented foods, such as kimchi and sauerkraut, are excellent sources of insoluble fiber.

LUNCH

Add leftover rice, pasta, or potatoes to a salad for lunch. When these ingredients are cooked and cooled, some of the starch they contain becomes resistant starch. This means that they begin to act in the same way as prebiotic fiber, encouraging the growth of friendly bacteria.

DINNER

Diets that are high in saturated fat can disrupt the balance of bacteria in the gut. Choose healthy fats from avocados, nuts, and canola or olive oil and combine them with low-fat, protein-rich foods such as lean meat, poultry, fish, beans, legumes, or quinoa. Include plenty of vegetables in your meal to boost fiber.

Quinoa makes a meat-free, protein-rich base for your evening meal

Combine cooked brown rice with plenty of vegetables for a lunchtime salad

BARLEY

Containing more fiber than any other whole grain, as well as very high levels of selenium, barley helps maintain digestive health and may protect against cancer.

WHY EAT IT?

HEART HEALTH
Beta-glucan is a form of fiber that is found in high quantities in barley, especially in whole-grain hulled barley. Research has shown that beta-glucan can help reduce bad cholesterol and a type of fat called triglycerides, helping protect against heart disease.

DIGESTIVE HEALTH
Barley contains more fiber than any other whole grain. This is a mixture of soluble and insoluble fiber, which helps speed the passage of waste material through your digestive tract and encourages the growth of gut-friendly bacteria.

CANCER PREVENTION
Barley is an excellent source of the mineral selenium, which nutritional surveys show is lacking in many people's diets. Research shows that selenium may help reduce the risk of cancer.

WHAT'S IN IT?

A 1-cup serving of cooked hulled barley provides a great source of selenium, vitamin B1, beta-glucan, and magnesium. Barley also contains protein, iron, and zinc.

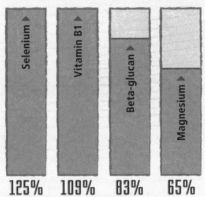

Selenium	Vitamin B1	Beta-glucan	Magnesium
125%	109%	83%	65%

Percentage of your daily reference intake

WHERE IS IT FROM?

Cultivated as early as 8000 BCE, barley is now one of the most widely grown crops in the world. The kernels of the plant are used for food or to make beer.

Barley is ready to harvest when the kernels are fully formed and firm

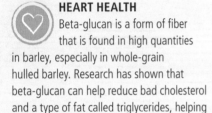
Choose hulled barley, rather than pearl barley, as it retains its fiber-rich husk

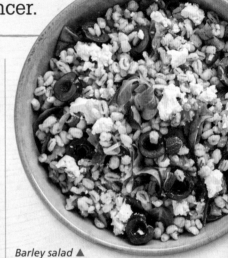
Barley salad ▲

HOW TO EAT IT

1 BARLEY SALAD
For a simple, main course salad, combine cooked barley with halved cherries, goat cheese, walnuts, almonds, and salad leaves. Toss with a bright citrus dressing.

2 HEALTHIER RISOTTO
Replace Arborio rice with the nutritional powerhouse of barley in a risotto. Pair with portobello mushrooms to complement the dark, nutty flavor of the grain.

3 ADD TO STEWS
Bulk up a warming stew of chicken and root vegetables with barley. Blanch a large handful of barley before adding it to the stew.

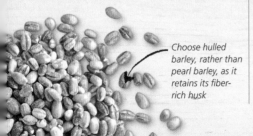

WHOLE-GRAIN RICE

Whole-grain rice, such as brown, red, and black rice, contains high levels of gut-friendly fiber and bone-strengthening manganese.

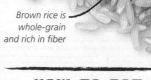

Brown rice is whole-grain and rich in fiber

WHY EAT IT?

 HEART HEALTH
Studies show that people who eat at least three servings of whole grains, such as brown, red, or black rice, each day are 30 percent less likely to suffer from heart disease, stroke, and type 2 diabetes.

 BONE STRENGTH
Whole-grain rice contains high quantities of manganese—studies have linked low manganese levels with an increased risk of osteoporosis.

 DIGESTIVE HEALTH
Containing almost three times more fiber than white rice, brown rice helps keep your gut healthy.

MAXIMIZE THE BENEFITS

TRY DIFFERENT VARIETIES
Black and red rice get their color from a group of phytochemicals called anthocyanins, which are believed to help keep your brain healthy.

WHAT'S IN IT?

A 1-cup serving of cooked brown rice provides good quantities of manganese, selenium, phosphorus, and magnesium. Brown rice also contains fiber.

Manganese	Selenium	Phosphorus	Magnesium
82%	33%	32%	23%

Percentage of your daily reference intake

WHERE IS IT FROM?

Rice is a type of grass that is grown across Asia in shallowly flooded paddy fields. Rice plants grow to 4ft (1.2m) in height.

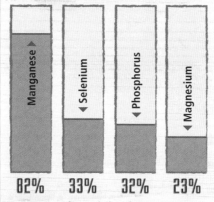

Rice grains are harvested from spiky flower heads

HOW TO EAT IT

1 BROWN RICE STIR-FRY
Cooked and cooled brown rice makes a flavorful, nutty base for a vegetable stir-fry packed with greens and seeds. Add it to the wok toward the end of cooking.

2 SIMPLE SUSHI
Turn leftover cooked rice into a quick sushi roll for a nutritious lunch. Wrap the rice, sliced avocado, and julienned cucumber in nori sheets and sprinkle with black sesame seeds.

3 IN A SALAD
Dress cooked, cooled brown rice with a strong, citrus-based dressing, toss with plenty of chopped fresh herbs, and use as a base for a filling and nutritious salad.

BROWN RICE POWER BOWL

This satisfying meal-in-a-bowl is an excellent source of fiber, which supports a healthy digestive system. Sweet potatoes are rich in immune-boosting vitamin C, while kale helps maintain healthy bones.

Serves 1   **Prep time** 20 minutes   **Cook time** 30–40 minutes

INGREDIENTS

½ cup **brown rice**, preferably basmati

½ **sweet potato**, peeled and cut into ½in (1cm) dice, 4½oz (125g) prepared weight

1½ tbsp olive oil

salt and freshly ground black pepper

⅛oz (5g) dried **wakame**

1 large **egg**

1 tsp **sesame oil**

1 large handful **kale**, washed, deribbed, and finely shredded, about 1½oz (45g) prepared weight

1 tbsp reduced-sodium soy sauce

1 tbsp **pumpkin seeds**

METHOD

1 Preheat the oven to 400°F (200°C). Cook the rice in plenty of boiling, salted water until it is just al dente, according to the package instructions. Depending on the type, it should take between 20 and 30 minutes.

2 While the rice is cooking, toss the diced sweet potatoes in half a tablespoon of olive oil and place them in a single layer on a baking sheet. Season well and bake at the top of the oven for 20–25 minutes, turning them halfway through the cooking time.

3 Put the wakame in a small bowl and cover with hand-hot water from the tap. Soak it for 10–15 minutes, then drain it well and squeeze it dry in some paper towels. Remove any tough stalks from the seaweed and coarsely chop it.

4 When the rice is cooked, drain it. At the same time, fill a small pan with boiling water. Crack an egg into it carefully and poach it for 2–3 minutes until just set.

5 While the egg is cooking, heat the sesame oil in a wok, then add the kale and stir-fry for 1 minute, until it starts to wilt. Add the soy sauce and cook for another minute. Remove it from the wok. Add the cooked and strained rice, chopped wakame, and pumpkin seeds to the wok and turn them briefly through to combine all the ingredients.

6 Put the rice mixture into a bowl. Add the cooked sweet potatoes and kale to the top of the rice on one side, and then place the just-poached egg gently on top of the rice. Eat immediately.

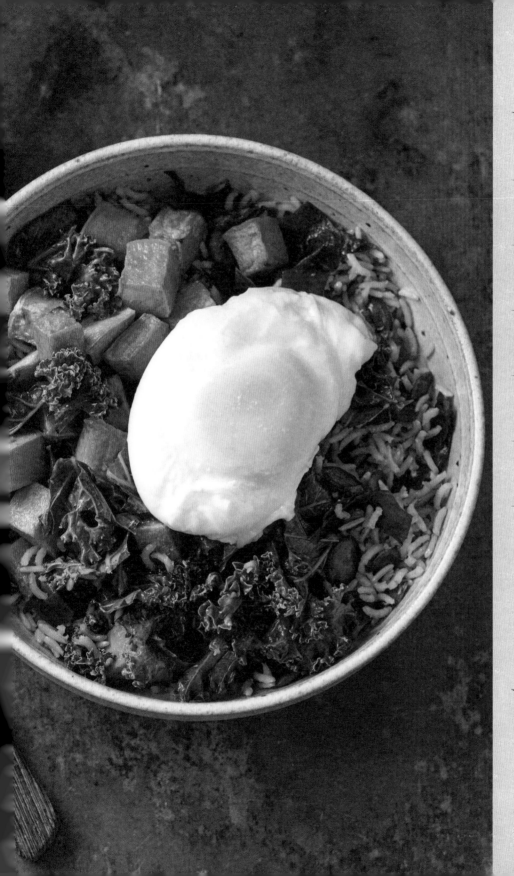

FEATURED SUPERFOODS

BROWN RICE
supports **digestive health**

SWEET POTATOES
help maintain your **immune system**

WAKAME
helps regulate your **hormones**

EGGS
help support your **immune system**

SESAME OIL
may help maintain **heart health**

KALE
helps keep your **bones healthy**

PUMPKIN SEEDS
are good for **skin health**

Nutrition per serving

Energy 870cals (3502kj)

Carbohydrate 104g
– of which sugars 8g

Fiber 13g

Fat 36g
– of which saturated 6g

Salt 2.2g

Protein 26g

Cholesterol 214g

QUINOA

Gluten-free quinoa is a complete protein—it contains all the essential amino acids—and helps your body grow and repair tissue. It also contains manganese, which supports your circulatory and nervous systems, and immune-boosting zinc.

WHY EAT IT?

BLOOD HEALTH

Iron is essential for the manufacture of red blood cells, which carry oxygen around the body. Quinoa contains three times more iron than brown rice, making it a great choice for those at risk of anemia—nutritional surveys show that 1 in 4 women under the age of 50 have low iron stores. Quinoa also contains folate, a B vitamin that helps your body produce healthy red blood cells, which may help to lower the risk of cardiovascular disease.

HIGH IN MANGANESE

The high levels of manganese in quinoa support many of the chemical processes that happen in your body, including energy production. Manganese also helps keep your blood, brain, and nerves healthy. Studies suggest that it may also help control blood sugar levels and prevent osteoporosis.

IMMUNE BOOST
Quinoa is a useful source of zinc, which is important for the body to maintain a healthy immune system. Since zinc is lost from the body through sweat, active people in particular benefit from a good dietary intake of zinc.

WHAT'S IN IT?

A 1-cup serving of cooked quinoa is a good source of manganese, folate, magnesium, and iron. Quinoa also contains vitamins B1, B2, B6, and E, as well as zinc, copper, phosphorus, potassium, and selenium.

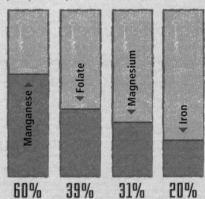

Manganese	Folate	Magnesium	Iron
60%	39%	31%	20%

Percentage of your daily reference intake

Quinoa contains **three times** more **iron** than brown rice, making it a **useful** food for those at **risk** of **anemia**.

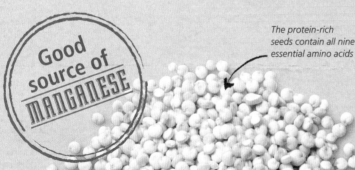

The protein-rich seeds contain all nine essential amino acids

Good source of MANGANESE

WHERE IS IT FROM?

Quinoa has been cultivated since about 3000 BCE. It is native to the Andean region of South America and was a sacred food of the Incas, who called it the mother grain. The main producing countries are Bolivia, Peru, and the United States. The grains are actually the edible seeds of a flowering plant.

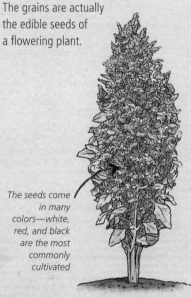

The seeds come in many colors—white, red, and black are the most commonly cultivated

MAXIMIZE THE BENEFITS

CHOOSE ALL COLORS
All varieties of quinoa are complete proteins. Red quinoa has the added antioxidant properties of the pigment betacyanin, and black quinoa contains high levels of gut-healthy fiber.

SPROUT IT
Sprout quinoa (see p67) to help your body access B vitamins in the grains.

HOW TO EAT IT

1 QUINOA OATMEAL
Try substituting your usual oats for quinoa. Cook over low heat with coconut or almond milk and top with honey, sliced almonds, and berries.

2 PATTIES
To make spicy falafel-inspired quinoa patties, mix cooked quinoa with ground cumin and cilantro, chopped parsley, and breadcrumbs, then bind the mixture with egg. Shape into patties and pan-fry until golden brown.

3 QUINOA VEGETABLE SOUP
Give a simple soup extra bulk and texture with added quinoa. Cook chopped onion, carrot, a rib of celery, and a clove of garlic until soft. Add a can of chopped tomatoes (with their juice), cooked quinoa, and seasoning, then simmer gently for 15 minutes until cooked. Process in a blender with some chopped parsley.

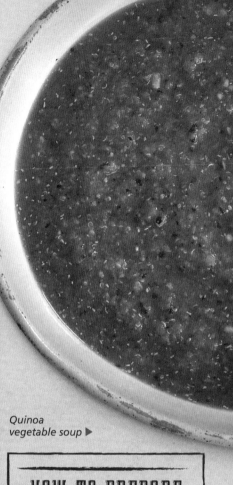

Quinoa vegetable soup ▶

TIP
Store cooked quinoa in an airtight container in the refrigerator for up to 5 days, or in the freezer for up to 2 months.

HOW TO PREPARE

To cook quinoa, first remove the bitter coating by washing the grains in a fine-mesh strainer. Boil for 10–15 minutes. The grains are ready when they have quadrupled in size and look translucent with a small "tail."

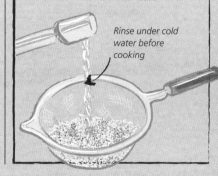

Rinse under cold water before cooking

QUINOA, CASHEW, & VEGETABLE STIR-FRY

Packed with protein and vitamin A, this bright stir-fry supports your immune system and helps keep your bones strong. Quinoa is a useful source of iron, which is essential for healthy blood and balanced energy levels.

Serves 2   **Prep time** 5 minutes   **Cook time** 25 minutes, plus cooling

INGREDIENTS

½ cup **quinoa**, rinsed

1 tsp reduced-sodium vegetable stock powder

¼ cup raw **cashews**

1 tbsp coconut oil

2 medium **carrots**, peeled and julienned, about 3½oz (100g) prepared weight

½ small red **onion**, finely sliced, about 2½oz (75g) prepared weight

1 cup bean sprouts

1½ cups Savoy **cabbage**, coarsely shredded

1 mild red or green chile, seeded and finely chopped

FOR THE SAUCE

1½in (3cm) piece of **ginger**, peeled and finely grated

1 large clove **garlic**, crushed

1 tbsp lime juice

1 scant tbsp honey

2 tbsp reduced-sodium soy sauce

1 tsp **sesame oil**

METHOD

1 Place the quinoa in a small, heavy-bottomed saucepan with the vegetable stock powder and 1 cup cold water. Bring to a boil, then reduce to a low simmer and cook, covered, for 15 minutes until all the liquid has been absorbed and the grains develop a "ring" around them, known as the germ.

2 Turn the cooked quinoa onto a large plate, fork through to separate the grains, and let cool. At this point, the quinoa can be refrigerated for up to 3 days before using.

3 To make the sauce, whisk all the ingredients together in a small bowl until combined. Set aside until needed.

4 Heat a wok over medium heat and dry-fry the chopped cashews for 2–3 minutes, stirring constantly, until they start to color in places and turn golden brown. Remove from the pan and coarsely chop.

5 Wipe the pan with a piece of paper towel to remove any nut residue (which will otherwise burn).

6 Heat the coconut oil over high heat until it starts to almost smoke. Add the carrots and stir-fry for 1 minute. Add the onion and cook for another minute. Finally, add the bean sprouts and cabbage and cook for another minute, along with the chile.

7 Add the sauce to the pan, mix it well, then add the cooled quinoa to the vegetables. Turn them through well and cook for a final 1–2 minutes until the quinoa is heated through. Scatter the cashews over the top of the dish and serve immediately.

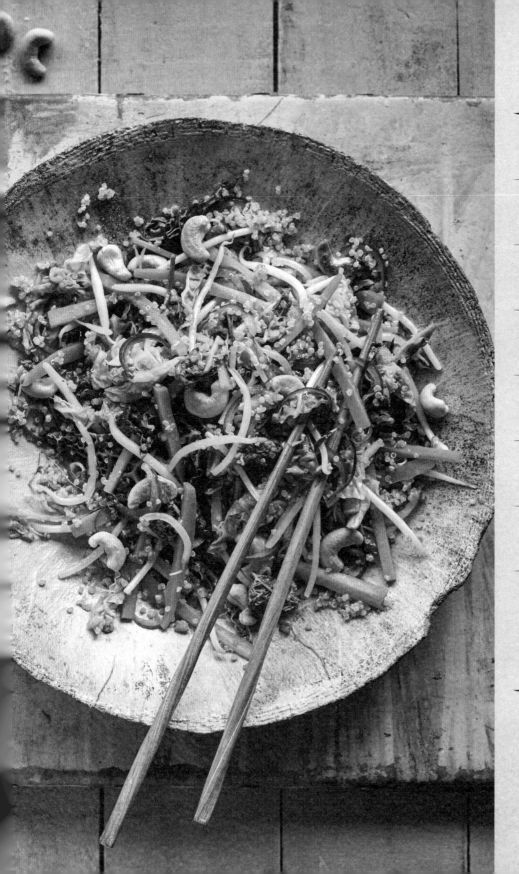

FEATURED SUPERFOODS

QUINOA
helps strengthen
your **bones**

CASHEWS
may help reduce
bad cholesterol

CARROTS
reduce the risk of certain
types of **cancer**

ONIONS
encourage the growth
of **gut-friendly bacteria**

CABBAGE
protects the cells that build
the **immune system**

GINGER
lowers the risk of
high blood pressure

GARLIC
may deactivate
cancer-causing agents

SESAME OIL
may help maintain
heart health

Nutrition per serving

Energy	418cals (1687kj)
Carbohydrate	48g
– of which sugars	20g
Fiber	9g
Fat	17g
– of which saturated	7g
Salt	1.5g
Protein	15g
Cholesterol	0g

AMARANTH

Gluten-free and whole-grain, amaranth seeds contain high levels of manganese, which helps your body produce energy. Amaranth also contains heart-healthy phytochemicals.

WHY EAT IT?

BLOOD HEALTH
Amaranth is a good source of iron, which is needed for the manufacture of hemoglobin—the red pigment in blood that carries oxygen around your body.

HEART HEALTH
Amaranth contains the phytochemicals rutin and nicotiflorin—antioxidants that are believed to help prevent cholesterol that can build up in blood vessels and restrict the flow of blood to the heart and brain.

BONE STRENGTH
Amaranth is rich in phosphorus, which works with calcium to help build strong bones and teeth.

The iron-rich seeds have a slightly peppery, nutty flavor and a sticky texture

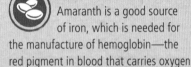

WHAT'S IN IT?

A 1-cup serving of cooked amaranth provides an excellent source of manganese, phosphorus, magnesium, and iron.

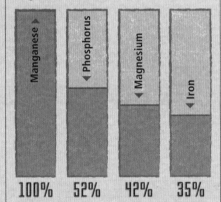

Manganese	Phosphorus	Magnesium	Iron
100%	52%	42%	35%

Percentage of your daily reference intake

WHERE IS IT FROM?

The Aztecs first cultivated amaranth around 8,000 years ago in what is now Mexico, and it is still a native crop in Peru. Amaranth is a bushy plant with tall, broad leaves and bright purple, red, or gold flowers. Amaranth seeds are tiny—about the same size as poppy seeds—and plants can produce up to 500,000 seeds per harvest.

HOW TO EAT IT

1 WHEAT-FREE TABBOULEH
Use this ancient grain to create a wheat-free tabbouleh. Replace bulgur wheat with cooked and cooled amaranth, and finish with handfuls of fresh herbs.

2 IN A PILAF
Add a deep, nutty complexity to amaranth by toasting it in a little olive oil over low heat until golden brown, and then use it as a base for a pilaf.

3 ADD TO SOUP
Add a couple of tablespoons of amaranth to a broth and allow it to thicken as it cooks.

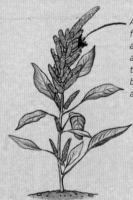

After the flowers of the amaranth plant are harvested, they are dried before the seeds are removed

BUCKWHEAT

Rich in soluble and insoluble fiber, copper, manganese, and magnesium, buckwheat supports your gut, bone, and blood health.

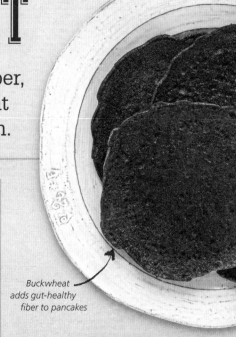

Buckwheat adds gut-healthy fiber to pancakes

Buckwheat pancakes ▲

WHY EAT IT?

DIGESTIVE HEALTH
Buckwheat is a useful source of insoluble fiber—this speeds up the passage of waste material through the digestive tract and helps to prevent constipation and diverticular disease. One type of starch also helps stimulate the growth of "friendly" bacteria in the gut.

HEART HEALTH
Buckwheat is a good source of soluble fiber, which, after digestion, forms a thick gel that binds to excess cholesterol and prevents it from being absorbed into the blood.

BLOOD HEALTH
Buckwheat converts into sugar slowly. This produces a slow, steady rise in blood sugar levels, rather than a sudden spike. Buckwheat also contains the phytochemical rutin that can help to lower blood pressure.

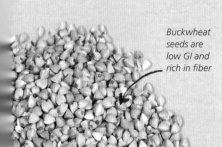

Buckwheat seeds are low GI and rich in fiber

WHAT'S IN IT?

A 1-cup serving of buckwheat is an excellent source of copper, manganese, magnesium, and fiber. It also contains folate, vitamins B1 and B2, iron, and phosphorus.

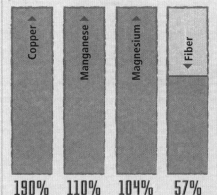

Copper	Manganese	Magnesium	Fiber
190%	110%	104%	57%

Percentage of your daily reference intake

WHERE IS IT FROM?

First cultivated in Southeast Asia in around 6000 BCE, buckwheat is a plant related to rhubarb, sorrel, and knotweed.

The plant has a growing period of 10–12 weeks

HOW TO EAT IT

1 BUCKWHEAT PANCAKES
Buckwheat flour is traditionally used to make all kinds of *crêpes* and pancakes. Use it to replace normal flour and add buttermilk for a healthy breakfast pancake, topped with honey and sliced bananas.

2 SPRINKLE ON SOUP
Top a rich, earthy borscht with its traditional accompaniment of sour cream and dill, and finish with a sprinkle of cooked buckwheat for added texture.

3 SOBA NOODLES
Good-quality soba noodles are made with 100 percent buckwheat flour. Seek them out in Asian supermarkets, and use them to make ramen or a classic soba noodle salad, dressed with sesame oil.

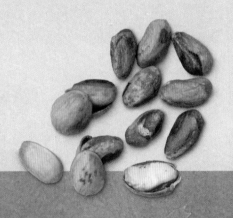

NUTS
& SEEDS

ALMONDS

Containing more protein, fiber, vitamin E, and calcium than other nuts, almonds may reduce the risk of heart disease, keep your bones healthy, and help your body absorb essential nutrients.

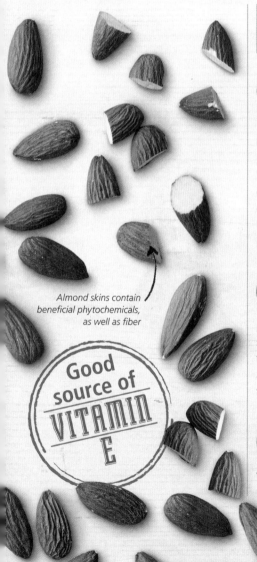

Almond skins contain beneficial phytochemicals, as well as fiber

Good source of **VITAMIN E**

WHY EAT IT?

HEART HEALTH
Almonds contain several phytochemicals, including beta-sitosterol, stigmasterol, and campesterol, that are believed to help reduce the risk of heart disease. Studies show that eating just a handful of almonds a day, as part of a low-fat diet and active lifestyle, may help to reduce levels of bad cholesterol in the blood by up to 10 percent.

BONE STRENGTH
Almonds are a useful source of calcium, particularly for people who do not eat dairy. Studies suggest that almonds may also help lower the risk of osteoporosis by reducing the activity of osteoclasts—cells that stimulate the loss of calcium from your bones.

SKIN HEALTH
Almonds are rich in vitamin E, a powerful antioxidant that helps to protect the skin from damage by free radicals. Essential fatty acids in almonds can also help to improve skin elasticity.

WHAT'S IN IT?

A 3-tablespoon serving of almonds is a good source of vitamin E, biotin, magnesium, and calcium. Almonds also contain vitamins B1, B2, and B6, as well as protein, fiber, folate, phosphorus, iron, zinc, copper, and manganese.

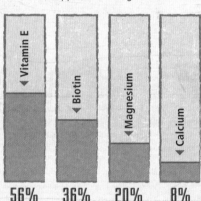

Vitamin E	Biotin	Magnesium	Calcium
56%	36%	20%	8%

Percentage of your daily reference intake

Eating just a **handful** of almonds **every day** may **reduce** levels of **bad cholesterol** by up to **10 percent**.

WHERE IS IT FROM?

The almond tree is native to Southwest Asia, and is now cultivated in the U.S., Europe, the Middle East, and Australia. Almonds are mentioned in the Bible, and were being eaten as a snack by Silk Road travelers by the first century CE. They are technically a fruit rather than a nut, as the seeds are contained within a shell and surrounded by fleshy fruit, making them botanically similar to walnuts and pecans.

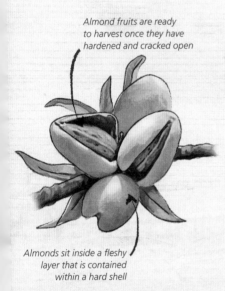

Almond fruits are ready to harvest once they have hardened and cracked open

Almonds sit inside a fleshy layer that is contained within a hard shell

MAXIMIZE THE BENEFITS

CHOOSE UNBLANCHED ALMONDS

Many of the phytochemicals and much of the fiber in almonds is found in the skin, so choose unblanched, raw almonds for maximum health benefits. Blanched almonds have had their nutritious layer removed.

TIP

Almonds contain fats that go rancid over time, so store them in an airtight container in a cool, dark place, and use as soon as possible.

HOW TO EAT IT

1 NUT BUTTER

A tasty alternative to peanut butter, almond butter is easy to make at home. Simply grind skin-on almonds in a high-powered food processor—it may take up to 20 minutes to get a creamy texture. Scrape the mixture down the sides of the bowl as you go.

2 ALMOND MILK

Homemade almond milk is a super-smooth, creamy drink that makes delicious smoothies. Soak almonds in water overnight, then rinse and blend with fresh water and filter through a cheesecloth to remove the almond meal.

3 YOGURT AND ALMOND BREAKFAST PARFAIT

Almonds are a good source of energy and protein, and a great way to start the day. Layer them up with plenty of fresh fruit and yogurt for a simple breakfast parfait.

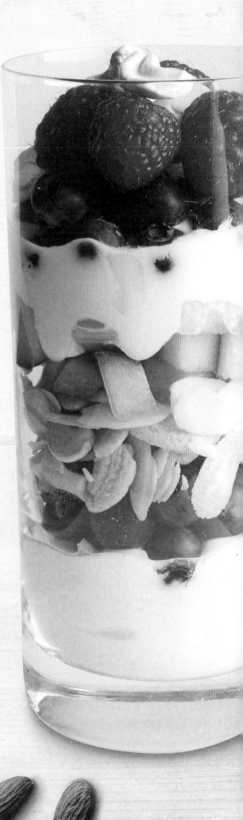

Yogurt and almond breakfast parfait ▶

PISTACHIOS

Rich in monounsaturated fats and potassium, pistachios help reduce levels of bad cholesterol and reduce high blood pressure. The copper in pistachios supports healthy bones and blood, while antioxidant phytochemicals protect your eye health.

WHY EAT IT?

HEART HEALTH
Most of the fat in pistachios is monounsaturated fat, which can help reduce levels of bad cholesterol in your blood, reducing the risk of heart disease and stroke. They also contain phytosterols, which help maintain normal cholesterol and lower high cholesterol levels, helping reduce the risk of heart disease.

EYE HEALTH
Pistachios contain the phytochemicals lutein and zeaxanthin. These antioxidants help to protect your eyes from damage by free radicals and reduce the risk of age-related macular degeneration (AMD), which is the most common cause of loss of vision in older people.

BLOOD HEALTH
Pistachios contain more potassium than other nuts—one ¼-cup serving contains as much potassium as half a large banana. Potassium works to support blood health by counteracting the negative effects of sodium on blood pressure, helping your kidneys filter your blood efficiently. Diets rich in potassium may help control blood pressure.

Phytochemicals in pistachios help **protect** your **eyes** from **damage** by free radicals and **reduce** the risk of **age-related macular degeneration**.

WHAT'S IN IT?

A ¼-cup serving of pistachios provides a good source of copper, vitamin B6, potassium, and protein. Pistachios also contain vitamins A, E, and B1, as well as folate, magnesium, selenium, calcium, and fiber.

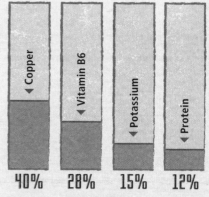

Copper	Vitamin B6	Potassium	Protein
40%	28%	15%	12%

Percentage of your daily reference intake

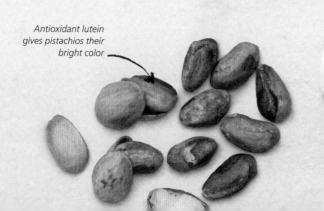

Antioxidant lutein gives pistachios their bright color

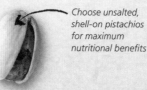

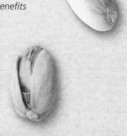

Choose unsalted, shell-on pistachios for maximum nutritional benefits

WHERE IS IT FROM?

Originating from Central Asia and the Middle East, the pistachio plant was cultivated as early as the Bronze Age. Related to the cashew family, the plant grows best in dry regions of the world, and is usually harvested in the fall. The fruits have a hard exterior that encloses the nuts.

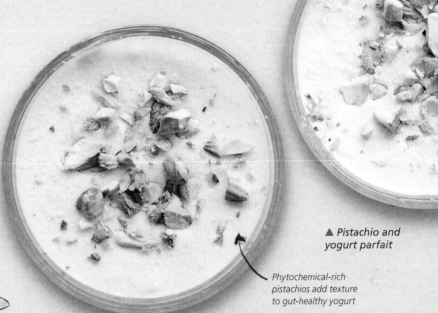

▲ Pistachio and yogurt parfait

Phytochemical-rich pistachios add texture to gut-healthy yogurt

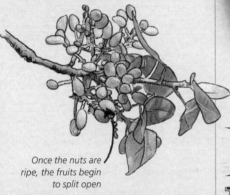

Once the nuts are ripe, the fruits begin to split open

MAXIMIZE THE BENEFITS

CHOOSE UNSHELLED NUTS
Since pistachios are high in fat, albeit mainly good fats, it's best to eat them in small quantities. Studies show that the process of opening pistachio shells slows down the rate at which you eat them and helps you feel fuller quicker. The pile of shells also acts as a visual reminder of how many you've eaten. Unshelled pistachios also remain fresh for longer, helping maintain nutrient levels.

CHOOSE UNSALTED
Added salt increases the quantity of sodium in your blood, which affects your kidneys' ability to filter your blood and maintain steady blood pressure.

HOW TO EAT IT

1 PISTACHIO AND YOGURT PARFAIT
If you have an ice-cream maker, it's simple to conjure up this healthy dessert. Simply mix plain Greek yogurt with a little honey, some orange-flower water, and a handful of chopped pistachios, and then freeze according to the machine instructions.

2 TOASTED SNACK
To make a healthy snack, dry-fry shelled pistachios until golden; add a drizzle of canola oil, spices, and a little honey; and cook for a couple more minutes until they are well glazed. Let cool before serving.

3 PISTACHIO PESTO
Make a simple pesto using toasted pistachios, arugula, garlic, lemon zest, and olive oil. You could also add a handful of freshly grated Parmesan cheese.

Pistachios contain **monounsaturated fat** and **phytosterols**, which help **reduce** levels of **bad cholesterol**.

TIP
Store unshelled pistachios in an airtight container in the fridge for up to 3 months. Eat shelled pistachios as quickly as possible.

CASHEWS

A rich source of healthy fats that help protect against heart disease, cashews also provide minerals, such as copper, manganese, and magnesium, that are good for bone health and support a host of chemical processes in the body.

WHY EAT IT?

HEART HEALTH
The high levels of monounsaturated fats found in cashews may help reduce bad LDL cholesterol when eaten regularly as part of a healthy diet. This helps lower the risk of heart disease and stroke.

BLOOD HEALTH
Cashews are rich in copper, which helps the body absorb and use iron, as well as helping your body make red and white blood cells. Cashews are also a useful source of iron for people who don't eat meat—iron helps your blood transport oxygen around the body.

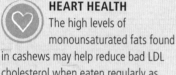

Good source of COPPER

BONE STRENGTH

As a good source of copper, cashews help build and maintain healthy bones and teeth, and may lower the risk of osteoporosis. Cashews also contain useful amounts of manganese, magnesium, and vitamin K, all of which are important for bone health.

Monounsaturated fats in cashews may help **reduce** levels of **bad cholesterol** in your blood, which can **lower** the **risk** of **heart disease**.

WHAT'S IN IT?

A ¼-cup serving of cashews provides a good source of copper, manganese, magnesium, and phosphorus. They also contain vitamins B1, B2, B6, E, and K, as well as iron, folate, selenium, potassium, zinc, protein, and fiber.

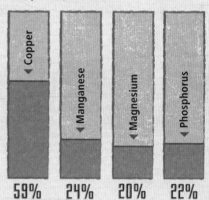

Copper	Manganese	Magnesium	Phosphorus
59%	24%	20%	22%

Percentage of your daily reference intake

Raw, unsalted cashews are the best choice if you are trying to avoid salt

WHERE IS IT FROM?

Originating from South America, cashews are the seeds of an evergreen tropical tree. The kidney-shaped "nuts" grow on the cashew apple (an edible stem rather than a true fruit), and have a double shell that is cracked before it is sold.

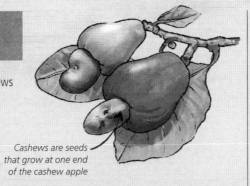

Cashews are seeds that grow at one end of the cashew apple

Cashews are a good source of **copper**, a mineral that helps **build** and **maintain** healthy **bones** and **teeth**, and may **reduce** the **risk** of developing **osteoporosis**.

HOW TO EAT IT

1 SPICED NUTS

Roasted, spiced cashews add flavor and crunch to even the simplest salad. Toss them in a little olive oil, honey, salt, and smoked paprika, then roast in a medium oven until golden brown.

2 DAIRY ALTERNATIVE

Cashew cream can be used whenever you need a sweetened cream. Soak the nuts overnight, then drain them and blend with water and a little honey to a thick, creamy consistency.

3 CASHEW AND CACAO BUTTER

Make your own, healthier version of a chocolate nut spread using cashews. Blend 2 cups of roasted cashews with 2 tablespoons of cacao nibs, ½ teaspoon of vanilla extract, and a little honey.

Cashew nut butter is great spread on toast or added to smoothies

TIP
The fat in cashews can become rancid if the nuts are stored too long, so buy small quantities and keep them in a cool, dark place.

Cashew and cacao butter ▶

RAW ENERGY BARS

These no-bake bars combine fiber-rich dried fruit with heart-healthy nuts and seeds. They contain a high quantity of copper, which supports the circulatory, skeletal, and nervous systems.

Makes 16 bars **Prep time** 20 minutes, plus chilling

INGREDIENTS

1 cup Medjool dates, pitted and coarsely chopped

1 cup dried apricots, coarsely chopped

½ cup dried **cherries** or **cranberries**, coarsely chopped

⅔ cup sliced **almonds**

⅔ cup raw **cashews**, coarsely chopped

½ cup **pumpkin seeds**

¼ cup **sunflower seeds**

½ cup coconut flakes

2 tbsp raw **cacao** powder

SPECIAL EQUIPMENT

8in (20cm) square baking pan
food processor

METHOD

1 Line the baking pan with parchment paper. Place the chopped dates in a heatproof bowl and cover with hot water. Let them soak while you prepare the rest of the ingredients.

2 After 5 minutes, drain the dates through a strainer. When cool enough to handle, press the dates lightly to remove some of the water, leaving them just a little damp. Place them in a food processor and add all the remaining ingredients.

3 Process the mixture until it is well combined, the nuts and seeds are in small pieces, and the mixture begins to form a ball in the bowl of the food processor. If the mixture is not blending thoroughly, take some out and process it in batches.

4 Dampen your hands and transfer the mixture to the lined baking pan. Push the mixture into an even layer using your hands. Dampen the back of a large metal spoon and use it to even out the surface of the mixture. Place the filled pan in the fridge for 3–4 hours.

5 Turn the mixture onto a cutting board and cut into 16 squares. Wrap the squares individually in wax paper to prevent them from sticking together, and store in an airtight container in the fridge until needed.

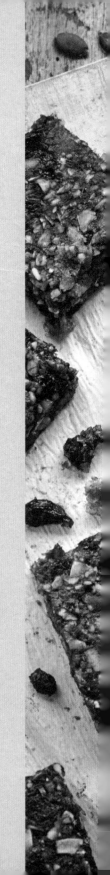

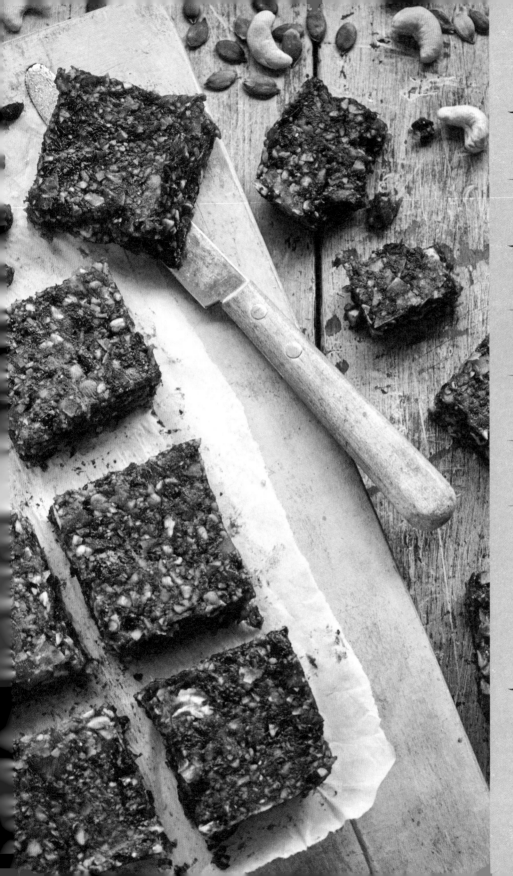

FEATURED SUPERFOODS

CHERRIES
may **improve** your **memory recall**

CRANBERRIES
prevent recurrent **urinary tract infections**

ALMONDS
reduce the risk of **heart disease**

CASHEWS
may help reduce **bad cholesterol**

PUMPKIN SEEDS
are good for **skin health**

SUNFLOWER SEEDS
help increase **good cholesterol**

CACAO
may help reduce the risk of **heart disease**

Nutrition per serving

Energy 150cals (598kj)
Carbohydrate 15g
– of which sugars 14g
Fiber 3g
Fat 7.5g
– of which saturated 2g
Salt 0g
Protein 4g
Cholesterol 0g

PINE NUTS

Pine nuts contain bone-strengthening vitamin K and antioxidant vitamin E. They are also extremely rich in manganese, which is needed for many of the chemical processes in your body.

WHY EAT IT?

BLOOD HEALTH
Pine nuts are a good source of vitamin K, which is important for the production of prothrombin, a protein that is essential for blood clotting.

BONE STRENGTH
The vitamin K in pine nuts helps your bones absorb calcium. Low levels of vitamin K in the blood are linked to a higher risk of osteoarthritis.

SKIN HEALTH
The vitamin E in pine nuts is a powerful antioxidant. It is an integral part of the skin's defense against UV radiation and other free radicals. Studies show that people with a low intake of vitamin E have an increased risk of developing cataracts.

Pine nuts are rich in free-radical-neutralizing vitamin E

WHAT'S IN IT?

A ¼-cup serving of pine nuts provides a good source of manganese, copper, and vitamins E and K. They also contain protein, zinc, magnesium, phosphorus, and iron.

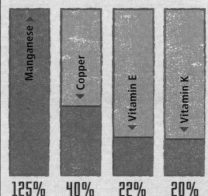

Manganese	Copper	Vitamin E	Vitamin K
125%	40%	22%	20%

Percentage of your daily reference intake

WHERE IS IT FROM?

Pine nuts are the edible seeds of pine trees. They grow in temperate regions around the world and have been harvested in Europe, North America, and Asia for thousands of years. The seeds develop under the scales of the pinecones and are released when the scales open.

HOW TO EAT IT

1 SUPERFOOD PESTO
Blend ½ cup of toasted pine nuts with a large handful of young kale, grated Parmesan cheese, a little garlic, and a drizzle of olive oil until combined.

2 ADD TO SALADS
Dry-fry pine nuts over low heat for a couple of minutes, stirring constantly, until golden brown. Cool and keep in an airtight container for sprinkling onto salads or rice dishes.

3 PINE NUT STUFFING
Mix low-fat ricotta with shredded spinach and toasted pine nuts for a quick and tasty stuffing for fish fillets or chicken breasts.

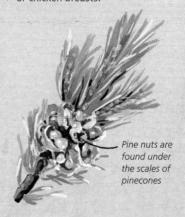

Pine nuts are found under the scales of pinecones

WALNUTS

Walnuts offer heart-friendly fats, immune-boosting copper, and manganese, which helps keep your brain and nerves healthy.

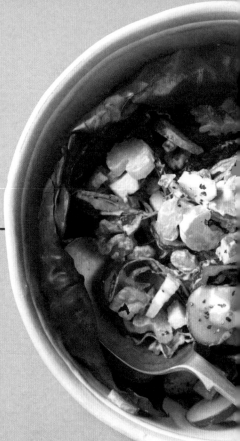

WHY EAT IT?

HEART HEALTH
What sets walnuts apart from other nuts is that they contain alpha-linolenic acid. This omega-3 fat can help lower the risk of heart disease by reducing high cholesterol levels and making your blood less likely to clot.

SKIN HEALTH
Essential fatty acids found in walnuts can help to strengthen the membranes of your skin cells, helping to lock in moisture and to keep skin looking radiant and youthful.

IMMUNE BOOST
Walnuts are a good source of copper, a trace element that plays an important role in the maintenance of your immune system. Copper helps in the manufacture of white blood cells.

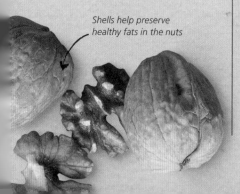

Shells help preserve healthy fats in the nuts

WHAT'S IN IT?

A ¼-cup serving of walnuts is a good source of manganese, copper, magnesium, and fiber. They also contain niacin, folate, and vitamins B1, B2, and E.

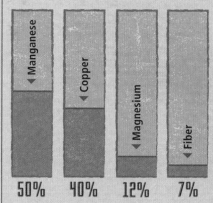

Manganese	Copper	Magnesium	Fiber
50%	40%	12%	7%

Percentage of your daily reference intake

WHERE IS IT FROM?

Dating back to 7000 BCE, walnuts are said to be the oldest tree food known to humankind. They are the seeds of the walnut tree and grow inside a husk.

A green, hairy husk contains the nut

Winter Waldorf salad ▲

HOW TO EAT IT

1 WINTER WALDORF SALAD
Combine toasted walnuts with celery, apples, red cabbage, radishes, and golden raisins for a nutrient-dense, Waldorf-style salad. Dress with yogurt and season with a little mustard, salt, and pepper.

2 FLAVOR DOUGH
Add ground walnuts to pie dough to complement fall fruit pie fillings, such as apples or pears. Process the walnuts gently with the flour until finely ground.

3 BAKE IN BREAD
Enhance simple, rustic soda bread with a few handfuls of chopped walnuts added into the dough before baking.

EATING FOR SLEEP

Getting enough sleep is vital for your health and well-being. Studies have shown that people who sleep for less than 6 hours each night have an increased risk of diabetes, heart disease, obesity, and early death. Here is an example of a day of eating to support a good night's sleep.

Keep hydrated with noncaffeinated drinks such as herbal tea

Yogurt is rich in melatonin-boosting calcium

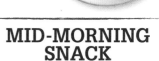

BREAKFAST

Choose a whole-grain, fortified breakfast cereal, or add wheatgerm to your oatmeal to increase your intake of B vitamins. Research has found that a deficiency of B vitamins, particularly B1, B6, and B12, can cause sleep problems, including insomnia and disrupted circadian rhythms.

TO DRINK

Drink caffeine-free liquids, such as water or herbal tea, throughout the day. It's especially important to avoid caffeinated drinks during the 6 hours before you go to bed. Coffee contains caffeine, as do most teas—including green tea—cola, and hot chocolate.

MID-MORNING SNACK

Eat yogurt halfway through the morning to top off your calcium levels. Calcium helps your brain manufacture the sleep hormone melatonin.

Choose breakfast cereals that are fortified with B vitamins

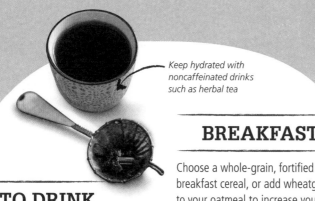

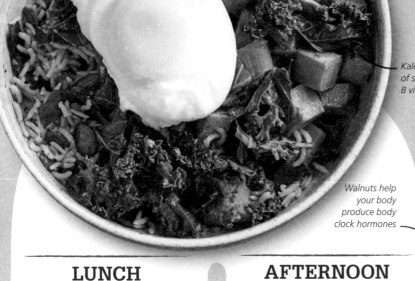

Kale is a good source of sleep-boosting B vitamins and iron

Walnuts help your body produce body clock hormones

Eat omega-3 fatty acids
Omega-3 fats, such as those found in oily fish, can help prevent sleep problems.

A little chopped bacon and fresh peas add protein to your evening meal

LUNCH

Restless leg syndrome, a constant urge to move the legs accompanied by a tingling sensation at night, affects as many as 1 in 10 people, and can disturb sleep. Scientists from the Sleep Disorder Unit at the New England Medical Center found that iron deficiency—even mild—may be responsible. Add iron-rich foods to your lunch, such as kale, lentils, and red meat.

AFTERNOON SNACK

Snack on almonds or walnuts to help set your body up for a good night's sleep. Almonds are a good source of magnesium, which helps the brain relax. Walnuts are rich in tryptophan, an essential amino acid that helps your body make serotonin and melatonin, the body clock hormones that control your body's sleep-wake cycle.

DINNER

A meal containing a small amount of protein and plenty of carbohydrates encourages your brain to produce the hormone serotonin, which will help you to feel relaxed and sleepy. Try to eat at least 3 hours before going to bed. Eating a heavy meal late in the evening causes your stomach to produce acid, which can result in heartburn and indigestion, interfering with the quality of your sleep.

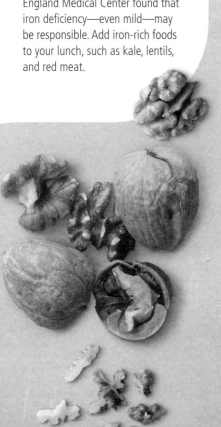

PEANUTS

Peanuts are higher in protein than most nuts and are full of vitamins. They also contain heart-healthy nutrients such as magnesium, niacin, copper, and oleic acid, and are a rich source of cancer-fighting resveratrol.

WHY EAT IT?

HEART HEALTH

The oleic acid in peanuts, as well as the protein and fiber, can help to lower bad LDL cholesterol while maintaining good levels of HDL cholesterol. *A New England Journal of Medicine* report has suggested that eating peanuts twice a week can reduce the risk of fatal heart disease by 24 percent.

BLOOD HEALTH

Peanuts are rich in the amino acid arginine, which can help to open up blood vessels, improving blood flow.

DISEASE PREVENTION

Peanuts are rich in a phytochemical called resveratrol, which is believed to help reduce the risk of certain types of cancer. It inhibits the growth of tumors by cutting off blood supply to the cells. Eating peanuts regularly has also been shown to help lower the risk of stroke.

WHAT'S IN IT?

A ¼-cup serving of unsalted peanuts provides a good source of copper, vitamin B1, niacin, and vitamin E. Peanuts also contain vitamins B2 and B6, as well as folate, potassium, phosphorus, magnesium, iron, zinc, protein, fiber, and manganese.

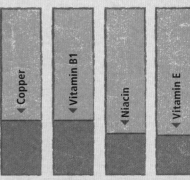

Copper	Vitamin B1	Niacin	Vitamin E
29%	29%	24%	24%

Percentage of your daily reference intake

Eating a portion of peanuts **twice weekly** has been shown to reduce the **risk of heart disease** by **24%**.

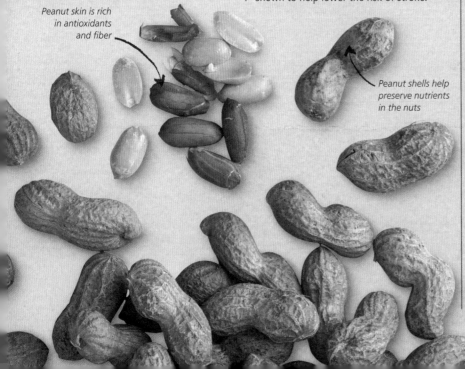

Peanut skin is rich in antioxidants and fiber

Peanut shells help preserve nutrients in the nuts

WHERE IS IT FROM?

A peanut is actually the seed of a plant in the legume family, originating in Central and South America. Today, peanuts are farmed in China, Indonesia, North America, and Nigeria, as well as many other countries. Each wrinkled shell contains one to four peanuts, individually wrapped in a thin, papery skin.

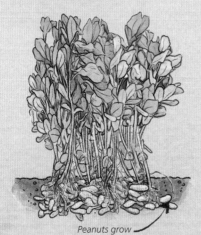

Peanuts grow beneath the soil, so are also known as groundnuts

MAXIMIZE THE BENEFITS

BUY UNSHELLED OR WITH SKIN ON
Since the shells keep the nutrients intact, unshelled peanuts (with intact outer shells) are best. They are available in airtight packs. If you do buy shelled, the skins contain high levels of phytochemicals and fiber, so choose those with their skin on. Avoid salted peanuts, as salt increases your blood pressure and can lead to stroke or heart disease.

HOW TO EAT IT

1 NUT BUTTER
Peanut butter is a great source of protein and healthy fats. Avoid the added sugar and salt by grinding your own in a food processor.

2 PEANUT SOUP
Peanut soup is a staple dish of West Africa. Cook red bell peppers, garlic, and onions with canned tomatoes and additive-free peanut butter until cooked through. Serve with brown rice.

3 THAI RED CURRY
Peanuts are often used as a thickener in African or Asian dishes, as well as for a salty, crunchy garnish. Add coarsely ground peanuts to a Thai red curry for a protein boost.

Thai red curry ▶

Peanuts are rich in the phytochemical **resveratrol**, which reduces the risk of some **cancers** by cutting off the blood supply to cancer cells.

TIP
Peanuts are best eaten as soon as possible. They last 3 months when stored in the fridge in an airtight container, or 1 year in the freezer.

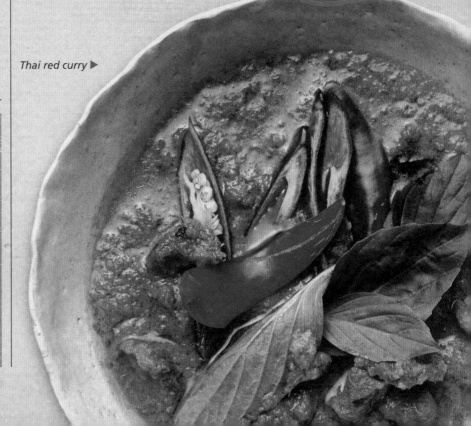

BRAZIL NUTS

Like all nuts, Brazils contain essential fatty acids and protein, but their superfood status is due to high levels of selenium. Just four nuts will provide over 100 percent of the recommended daily amount of this disease-fighting mineral.

WHY EAT IT?

DISEASE PREVENTION

Selenium is a powerful antioxidant, and people who do not get enough selenium in their diet may have an increased risk of some types of cancer. Selenium is also thought to help reduce the risk of cardiovascular disease and strengthen the immune system.

SKIN HEALTH

Selenium in Brazil nuts helps to protect the skin from damage by free radicals, which accelerate wrinkling and other signs of aging. In addition, it acts as an internal sunscreen, helping to protect the skin from inflammation caused by too much sun. It can be also effective for treating acne.

Buy Brazil nuts in their tough shells, which help preserve nutrients

HIGH IN COPPER

Copper helps the body absorb iron and use it to make red blood cells. It also helps to keep the blood vessels and immune system healthy, encourages the development of healthy bones and teeth, and maintains the myelin sheath around nerve fibers.

Brazil nuts are rich in **copper**, which helps your body manufacture **red blood cells** and maintain **blood vessels**.

Brazil nut skins are rich in fiber and antioxidants

WHAT'S IN IT?

A ¼-cup serving of Brazil nuts provides a great source of selenium, as well as high quantities of copper, magnesium, and vitamin E. Brazil nuts also contain vitamins B1 and B6, as well as folate, potassium, calcium, phosphorus, iron, zinc, and manganese.

Selenium	Copper	Magnesium	Vitamin E
129%	49%	31%	17%

Percentage of your daily reference intake

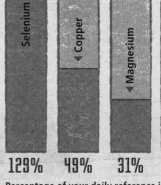

Great source of SELENIUM

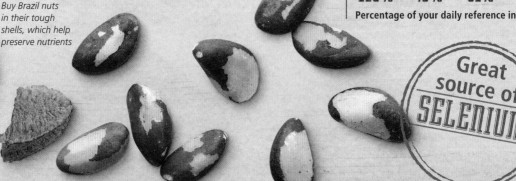

The exceptional levels of **selenium** in Brazil nuts are thought to decrease the risk of some types of **cancer**, as well as of **cardiovascular disease**. Selenium also strengthens the **immune system** and helps to protect the **skin** from signs of **aging**.

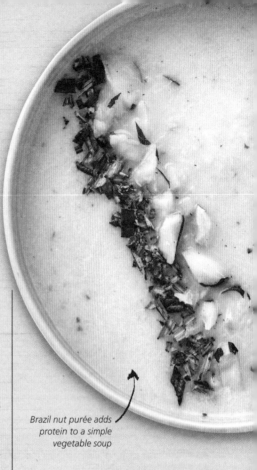

Brazil nut purée adds protein to a simple vegetable soup

Cauliflower and Brazil nut soup ▲

WHERE IS IT FROM?

Native to South America, Brazil nuts are the seeds of a tall tree that grows to a height of up to 160ft (50m) in the Amazon rainforest and can live for over 500 years. The trunk is erect, with a wide umbrella-like foliage near the top. The tree has not been successfully cultivated commercially, and the nuts are gathered mainly from the wild in Bolivia and Brazil for export, with smaller quantities coming from Peru. Each tree bears about 300 fruit pods in one season.

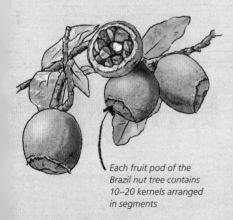

Each fruit pod of the Brazil nut tree contains 10–20 kernels arranged in segments

TIP

Brazil nuts should be firm when you bite into them, with a buttery texture on chewing. Avoid rubbery nuts and any that give off even a slightly rancid smell.

HOW TO EAT IT

1 CAULIFLOWER AND BRAZIL NUT SOUP

Brazil nuts have a wonderfully creamy texture, and a small handful of the skinned nuts puréed into a simple roasted cauliflower soup provides an added protein boost to a healthy lunch.

2 PESTO

Use toasted, chopped Brazil nuts in a basic recipe for pesto instead of the more usual pine nuts. Blend the nuts with large handfuls of basil, a little garlic, olive oil, and some grated Parmesan cheese.

3 IN BAKING

Ground Brazil nuts make a good substitute for ground almonds in gluten-free baking recipes. Grind them in a food processor, pulsing gently at the end to avoid overprocessing.

MAXIMIZE THE BENEFITS

BUY UNSHELLED
Brazil nuts contain high levels of polyunsaturated fats, which means they can become rancid quickly, so it is best to buy them unshelled. They will keep for a few months in a cool, dry place.

REFRIGERATE OR FREEZE SHELLED
If you do buy shelled Brazils, buy small quantities and store them in air-sealed bags in the fridge or freezer to preserve beneficial fats.

GLUTEN-FREE BRAZIL NUT BROWNIES

These brownies are based on ground Brazil nuts, which are rich in the cancer-fighting mineral selenium. Use dark chocolate, due to its high percentage of antioxidant-rich cacao, as it may help combat high blood pressure.

Makes 16 brownies   **Prep time** 20 minutes   **Cook time** 20–25 minutes

INGREDIENTS

3½oz (100g) good-quality, gluten-free dark chocolate

1½ cups shelled **Brazil nuts**, finely chopped

½ cup light brown sugar

5 tbsp cold unsalted butter, diced

4 extra-large **eggs**, separated

½ cup dried **cherries**, coarsely chopped

cacao powder, to serve

matcha powder, to serve (optional)

SPECIAL EQUIPMENT

8in (20cm) square brownie pan
food processor

METHOD

1 Preheat the oven to 350°F (180°C). Grease and line the brownie pan and set aside until needed.

2 Melt the chocolate in a bowl over a little simmering water, making sure that the bowl does not touch the water. Alternatively, carefully melt the chocolate in short bursts in a microwave on a low setting. Let the chocolate cool slightly.

3 In a food processor, grind 1 cup of the Brazil nuts with the sugar until the nuts are as fine as possible. Pulse toward the end, being careful not to overprocess the nuts, as this causes them to release their natural oils.

4 Add the butter and pulse until well combined, making sure not to overblend the mixture. With the processor running, add the egg yolks one at a time until they are completely mixed in. Finally, add the cooled chocolate and blend thoroughly.

5 In a separate bowl, whisk the egg whites to stiff peaks. Turn the brownie batter out of the food processor into a large bowl and beat in a few tablespoons of the egg whites to loosen the mixture. Gently fold in the remaining egg whites.

6 Gently fold in the remaining Brazil nuts and cherries and turn the batter into the prepared pan. Tip the pan gently from side to side to fill the corners and level the batter.

7 Bake in the center of the oven for 20–25 minutes, until a toothpick inserted into the middle of the brownie comes out partially clean. Remove from the oven and let cool in the pan for 10 minutes before turning onto a wire rack.

8 Let the brownie cool completely before peeling off the wax paper and slicing. To serve, dust with cacao powder and a little matcha powder, if using.

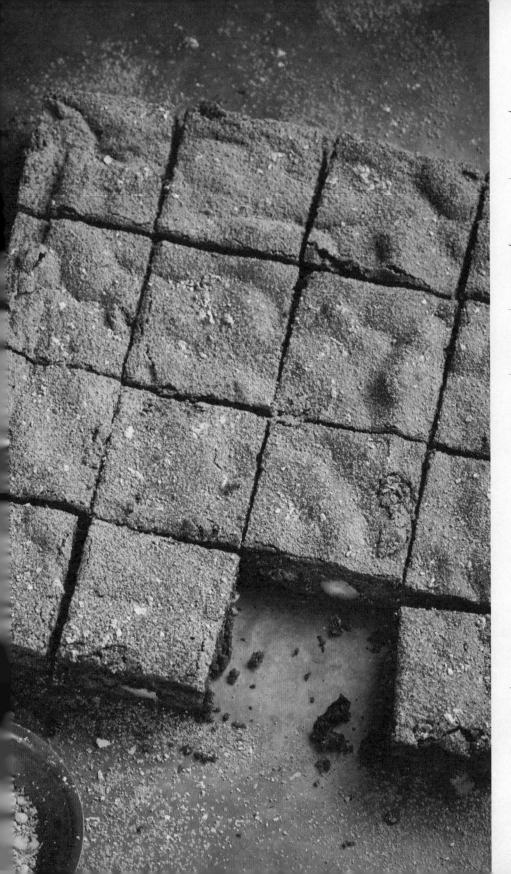

FEATURED SUPERFOODS

BRAZIL NUTS
may reduce the risk of
certain types of **cancer**

EGGS
help maintain a strong
immune system

CHERRIES
may improve your
memory recall

CACAO
may help reduce the risk
of **heart disease**

MATCHA POWDER
helps keep your
brain alert

Nutrition
per serving

Energy 220cals (901kj)
Carbohydrate 14g
– of which sugars 14g
Fiber 1g
Fat 16g
– of which saturated 6g
Salt 0.1g
Protein 5g
Cholesterol 72g

PUMPKIN SEEDS

Pumpkin seeds are a good source of zinc, which helps keep your skin and immune system healthy. They also contain magnesium, which supports skeletal and circulatory health.

WHY EAT IT?

IMMUNE BOOST
Pumpkin seeds are a good source of zinc, which helps to keep your immune system strong by boosting the production of cells that fight bacteria and viruses and inhibiting the growth of bacteria in your body.

SKIN HEALTH
Zinc is a vital mineral for growth and wound healing—it helps your skin to heal fast and maintains healthy skin. Some studies show that people with acne often have low levels of zinc in their blood.

WHAT'S IN IT?

A ½-cup serving of pumpkin seeds provides a good quantity of zinc, magnesium, iron, and protein. Pumpkin seeds also contain vitamins B1 and B2.

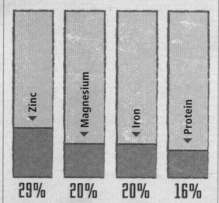

Zinc	Magnesium	Iron	Protein
29%	20%	20%	16%

Percentage of your daily reference intake

◀ Smoothie bowl

HOW TO EAT IT

1 AS A SNACK
Prepare fresh pumpkin seeds by removing them from a pumpkin and drying them. Toss them in a little oil and spices, and roast until golden brown.

2 PUMPKIN SEED MUFFINS
Try adding a handful of pumpkin seeds to a whole-wheat carrot muffin recipe for added texture and protein.

3 SMOOTHIE BOWL
Grind pumpkin seeds and add to smoothies, or simply sprinkle some seeds on top to provide a textural contrast to creamy smoothies.

WHERE IS IT FROM?

Pumpkin seeds are found in the central cavities of pumpkins. Native to Mexico, pumpkins are now widely grown as a field vegetable crop.

The seeds are scooped out and separated from the fibers

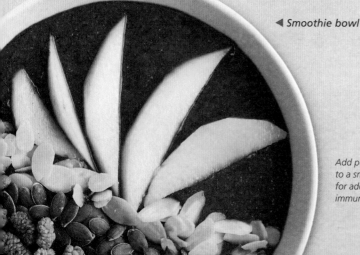

Add pumpkin seeds to a smoothie bowl for added texture and immune-boosting zinc

SUNFLOWER SEEDS

Sunflower seeds are an excellent source of vitamin E, which helps maintain healthy skin. They also contain oleic acid, which lowers bad cholesterol.

WHY EAT IT?

HEART HEALTH
Sunflower seeds contain high levels of monounsaturated fats, particularly oleic acid, which helps to keep the heart healthy by lowering bad LDL cholesterol and raising good HDL cholesterol.

SKIN HEALTH
Sunflower seeds are high in vitamin E, a powerful antioxidant that helps protect the skin against damage from free radicals, which can accelerate premature aging and wrinkles.

BLOOD HEALTH
The B vitamin folate, which is found in sunflower seeds, helps in the manufacture of red blood cells, keeping your blood healthy.

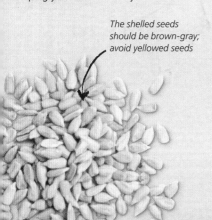

The shelled seeds should be brown-gray; avoid yellowed seeds

WHAT'S IN IT?

A ¼-cup serving of sunflower seeds provides a good source of vitamins E and B1, as well as folate and magnesium. Sunflower seeds also contain protein.

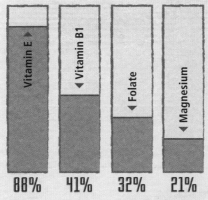

Vitamin E	Vitamin B1	Folate	Magnesium
88%	41%	32%	21%

Percentage of your daily reference intake

WHERE IS IT FROM?

Native to the southwestern part of North America, sunflowers are now cultivated in temperate regions, both for flowers and seeds. Fall is the season for sunflower seeds to be harvested. Depending on the variety, sunflower seeds have a black-and-white striped or black shell. The seeds are first dried before being sold shelled or unshelled.

HOW TO EAT IT

1 VEGAN MAYO
Blend sunflower seeds with water, garlic, and a little lemon juice, and season well to make an egg-free alternative to mayonnaise.

2 AS A SNACK
Eat a handful of sunflower seeds for a heart-healthy snack. Eat them raw, or season them with a little salt and roast in a medium oven until crisp.

3 COLESLAW CRUNCH
Sunflower seeds make an excellent addition to a fennel, cabbage, and apple 'slaw, along with a little oil and vinegar.

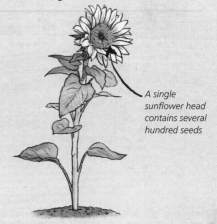

A single sunflower head contains several hundred seeds

CHIA SEEDS

Packed with fiber and essential fatty acids, chia seeds are also a good source of manganese and magnesium, which support healthy blood, nerves, and muscles.

WHY EAT IT?

DIGESTIVE HEALTH
Chia seeds are a good source of insoluble fiber, which helps to speed the passage of waste material through the digestive system, preventing constipation.

RICH IN MAGNESIUM
Magnesium, which is present in good quantities in chia seeds, helps support around 300 different chemical processes in your body. This vital mineral helps muscles relax, and keeps your heart and nervous system healthy.

HEART HEALTH
Chia seeds contain essential fatty acids, which are a source of omega-3 fatty acids. Omega-3 fatty acids protect against heart disease.

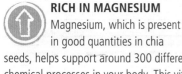

Chia seeds are mottled when ripe—avoid uniformly brown seeds, as these are unripe and contain fewer nutrients

WHAT'S IN IT?

A 2-tablespoon serving of chia seeds is a good source of manganese, magnesium, fiber, and phosphorus.

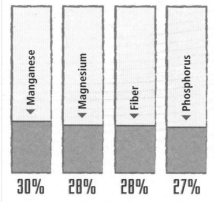

Manganese	Magnesium	Fiber	Phosphorus
30%	28%	28%	27%

Percentage of your daily reference intake

WHERE IS IT FROM?

Chia seeds come from a flowering plant in the mint family. Native to Central America, the plant was cultivated for its seeds as early as the Aztec period. It is now grown in Bolivia, Argentina, and Ecuador.

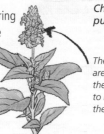

The flowers are dried and then crushed to release their seeds

HOW TO EAT IT

1 AS A TOPPING
Chia seeds can be added to homemade granola (see pp24–25) or sprinkled on top of any good-quality, store-bought granola or muesli.

2 IN CAKES AND BAKES
Try replacing poppy seeds with chia seeds in baked goods. Lemon and chia seed muffins, or banana and chia bread, make a delicious treat.

3 CHIA PUDDING
Combine chia seeds with yogurt, milk, and honey, and leave overnight in the fridge. Eat for breakfast with nuts and fruit.

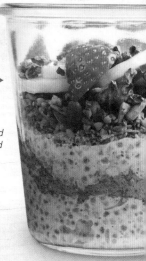

Chia pudding ▶

FLAXSEEDS

Flaxseeds, also known as linseeds, are a good source of the vital nutrients magnesium and manganese. They also contain omega-3 fatty acids and hormone-balancing phytochemicals.

WHY EAT IT?

♥ HEART HEALTH
Flaxseeds contain omega-3 fatty acids, which can help reduce the risk of heart disease. They work by preventing the formation of plaque that causes arteries to narrow.

⚖ HORMONE BALANCE
Phytochemicals called phytoestrogens are found in flaxseeds—these can help to reduce the incidence of hot flashes and other symptoms of the menopause.

MAXIMIZE THE BENEFITS

CRUSH THE SEEDS
Flaxseeds have tough cell walls, which make it difficult for your body to access their nutrients. To help your body digest the fiber-rich seeds, grind them in a coffee grinder or with a mortar and pestle before you use them. Whole flaxseeds stay fresh for longer than ground flaxseeds, so only grind a small quantity at a time and store any leftovers in the freezer.

WHAT'S IN IT?

A 2-tablespoon serving of flaxseeds is a good source of magnesium, manganese, vitamin B1, and fiber.

Magnesium	Manganese	Vitamin B1	Fiber
36%	35%	31%	25%

Percentage of your daily reference intake

WHERE IS IT FROM?

Flaxseeds were cultivated in the Middle East as early as 3000 BCE. The plants produce blue-purple flowers and grow to over 3¼ft (1m) tall.

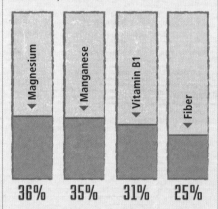

Flaxseeds are harvested from the flowers, and sold as they are or processed into oil

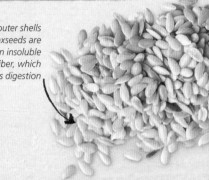

The outer shells of flaxseeds are rich in insoluble fiber, which aids digestion

HOW TO EAT IT

1 POWER POWDER
Boost your breakfast with a power powder. Simply grind flaxseeds with other superfoods, such as chia seeds and goji berries, and store in a jar. Add a tablespoon to your morning smoothie.

2 GLUTEN-FREE FLOUR
Flaxmeal is a good gluten-free substitute for ordinary flour. Grind your own in a powerful blender or coffee grinder and store in an airtight jar.

3 SUPERSEED MIX
Make a jar of superseed mix by mixing your favorite seeds such as flax-, chia, pumpkin, and sunflower seeds. Keep it handy as a last-minute addition to salads and sandwiches.

COCONUT & MANGO CHIA PUDDING

A deliciously creamy dessert or breakfast option, this pudding is based on magnesium- and fiber-rich chia seeds, which support your circulatory and nervous systems. Added mango offers cancer-fighting phytochemicals.

Serves 2   **Prep time** 5 minutes, plus overnight chilling

INGREDIENTS

flesh of 1 small **mango**, about ¾ cup chopped, plus extra, to serve

¾ cup reduced-fat coconut milk

3 tbsp **chia seeds**

1 tbsp honey

coconut flakes, toasted, to serve (optional)

SPECIAL EQUIPMENT

food processor or blender

METHOD

1 Place the mango and coconut milk in a food processor or blender and blend until smooth.

2 Add the chia seeds and honey and pulse briefly to combine. Place the mixture in a bowl, cover, and refrigerate overnight.

3 If the pudding is too thick the next day, loosen it with a little extra coconut milk until it reaches your desired consistency.

4 To serve, top the pudding with chopped fresh mango and toasted coconut flakes.

SUPER SWAP

Use vitamin E–rich almond milk in place of coconut milk, if you prefer. See p43 for a recipe for homemade almond milk.

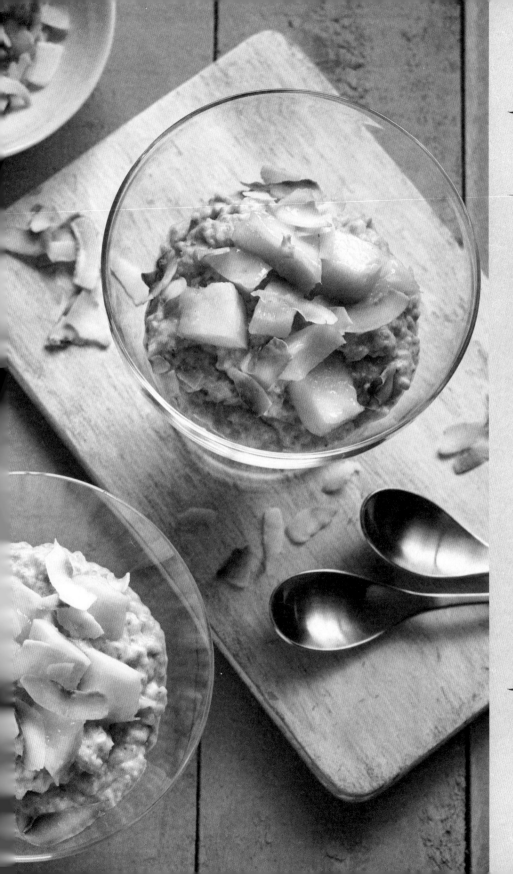

FEATURED SUPERFOODS

MANGO
may help reduce the
risk of certain types
of **cancer**

CHIA SEEDS
help keep your
heart and **nervous
system** healthy

Nutrition
per serving

Energy 228cals (877kj)
Carbohydrate 23g
– **of which sugars** 16g
Fiber 8g
Fat 12g
– **of which saturated** 7g
Salt 0g
Protein 3.5g
Cholesterol 0g

SESAME SEEDS

A useful source of copper, calcium, manganese, and phosphorus, sesame seeds help support circulatory, digestive, and skeletal health.

WHY EAT IT?

HEART HEALTH
Recent research suggests that sesame oil can reduce the level of triglycerides in the blood—this is a type of fat known to be associated with an increased risk of heart disease.

DIGESTIVE HEALTH
Sesame seeds contain phytochemicals called lignans, which slow the release of sugar into the blood and keep the digestive system healthy.

BONE STRENGTH
Sesame seeds can be a useful source of calcium for people who don't eat dairy. Research suggests that lignans present in sesame seeds may promote the growth of bone-forming cells called osteoblasts.

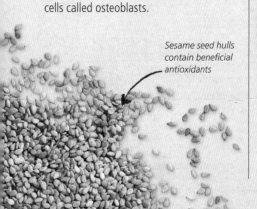

Sesame seed hulls contain beneficial antioxidants

WHAT'S IN IT?

A 1-tablespoon serving of sesame seeds is a useful source of copper, phosphorus, calcium, and manganese. Sesame seeds also contain vitamins B1, B6, and E, as well as niacin and folate.

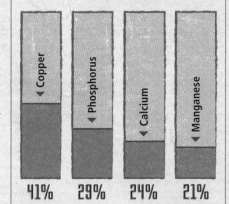

Copper	Phosphorus	Calcium	Manganese
41%	29%	24%	21%

Percentage of your daily reference intake

WHERE IS IT FROM?

The sesame plant is believed to originate from Asia or east Africa, and has been cultivated for its seeds for over 5,000 years.

Triangular pods contain the seeds

HOW TO EAT IT

1 HOMEMADE TAHINI
Tahini is a vital part of dishes such as hummus and falafel. Make your own by grinding sesame seeds with a little olive oil in a food processor.

2 SOY-GLAZED ROOT VEGETABLES
Turn all kinds of root vegetables into Asian-style sides by roasting them in a quick glaze of honey and soy sauce and sprinkling generously with sesame seeds.

3 SPICY FISH STICKS
Make homemade fish sticks by mixing panko breadcrumbs with sesame seeds and seasoning before lightly frying in a little sunflower oil.

MAXIMIZE THE BENEFITS

CHOOSE UNHULLED SEEDS
Black and brown sesame seeds have been found to have a higher antioxidant content than white seeds, which have had their hull removed.

ALFALFA SEEDS

Rich in cancer-fighting phytochemicals, alfalfa seeds are also a useful source of vitamin K, which supports blood health and helps keep your bones strong.

WHY EAT IT?

CANCER PREVENTION
Alfalfa seeds contain coumestans, which are part of a group of phytochemicals called phytoestrogens. This group may offer protection against different cancers, including breast cancer. Other studies have shown that they may help relieve some menopausal symptoms.

BONE STRENGTH
Vitamin K is present in useful quantities in alfalfa seeds. The vitamin is important for skeletal health, as it helps your bones absorb calcium.

BLOOD HEALTH
The folate in alfalfa seeds helps your body manufacture red blood cells, keeping your blood healthy.

WARNING
Under-5s, pregnant women, and elderly people should avoid eating sprouted alfalfa seeds.

WHAT'S IN IT?

A ¾-cup serving of sprouted alfalfa seeds is a useful source of vitamin K, folate, vitamin C, and magnesium.

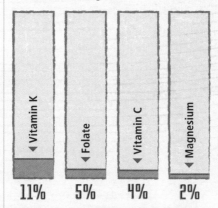

Vitamin K	Folate	Vitamin C	Magnesium
11%	5%	4%	2%

Percentage of your daily reference intake

WHERE IS IT FROM?

Part of the pea family, alfalfa was first cultivated in ancient Iran. Alfalfa flourishes in warmer-temperate climates and grows to 12–35in (30–90cm) tall.

Seeds are harvested from clusters of small, cloverlike flowers

HOW TO EAT IT

1 ALFALFA SPROUTS
Sprout your own alfalfa seeds using only a mason jar and a little cheesecloth. The seeds need to be first soaked, then rinsed frequently until the sprouts appear.

Alfalfa sprouts ▶

2 ADD TO SANDWICHES
Alfalfa sprouts make a great addition to any sandwich or wrap, adding crunch to smooth fillings, such as hummus or avocado.

3 IN TEA
Alfalfa tea has widespread uses in both Chinese and Ayurvedic medicine to treat a range of ailments. Steep dried leaves in boiling water for 5 minutes before straining.

Only choose alfalfa seeds that are labeled as edible, as these have been treated to eliminate bacteria

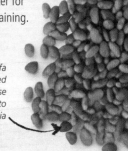

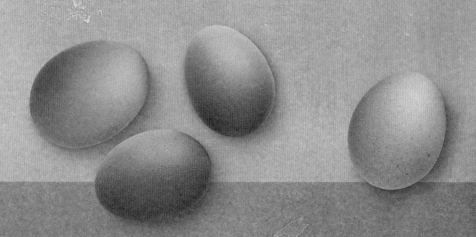

FISH, MEAT, DAIRY, & EGGS

OILY FISH

Oily fish, such as salmon, sardines, fresh tuna, and mackerel, are packed with blood-building vitamin B12, bone-strengthening vitamin D, and long-chain omega-3 fatty acids that can help keep your heart, brain, and skin healthy.

WHY EAT IT?

HEART HEALTH

 Oily fish provides the omega-3 fatty acids docosahexaenoic acid (DHA) and eicosapentaenoic acid (EPA), which are not found in many other foods. Omega-3 fatty acids are believed to lower the risk of heart disease and stroke by reducing levels of bad cholesterol in the blood, regulating your heartbeat, making the blood less likely to form clots that block blood flow, and lowering blood pressure. Studies show that eating at least two portions of oily fish per week lowers the risk of death from heart disease by 25 percent.

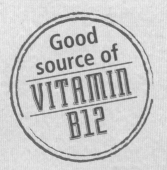

Good source of VITAMIN B12

BRAIN POWER

 Studies link low levels of DHA in the blood and brain with mental health problems such as depression and behavioral disorders. Other studies suggest a good intake of omega-3 fatty acids may reduce the risk of dementia and Alzheimer's disease later in life. These fats are especially important for pregnant women, as they support the growth of the baby's brain (see Warning, opposite).

SKIN HEALTH

Omega-3 fatty acids are thought to encourage the body to produce anti-inflammatory agents that help slow, and maybe even reverse, signs of aging such as wrinkles and loss of elasticity. Oily fish also provides protein, an essential ingredient of collagen, which keeps the skin firm. Omega-3 fatty acids can also help relieve symptoms associated with eczema and psoriasis.

A fresh mackerel will feel firm and have shiny skin and bright eyes

WHAT'S IN IT?

A 5½oz (150g) serving of wild salmon provides an excellent source of vitamins B12 and D, as well as omega-3 fatty acids DHA and EPA, and selenium. Salmon has one of the highest levels of omega-3 fatty acids of any oily fish.

Vitamin B12	Vitamin D	DHA/EPA	Selenium
392%	258%	86%	74%

Percentage of your daily reference intake

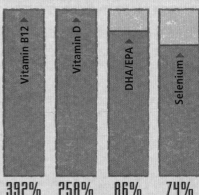

▲ *Mackerel*

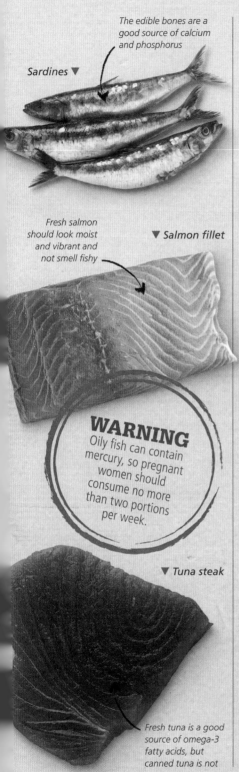

The edible bones are a good source of calcium and phosphorus

Sardines ▼

Fresh salmon should look moist and vibrant and not smell fishy

▼ **Salmon fillet**

WARNING
Oily fish can contain mercury, so pregnant women should consume no more than two portions per week.

▼ *Tuna steak*

Fresh tuna is a good source of omega-3 fatty acids, but canned tuna is not

HOW TO EAT IT

1 GRILL IT
Transform the flavor of salmon or mackerel by marinating it in a teriyaki sauce, then grilling it on both sides until the skin is crispy and golden brown.

2 FISHCAKES
For leftover grilled salmon or tuna, try making a quick and healthy fishcake. Mix cooked fish with baked and mashed sweet potato, scallions, and herbs, then coat in whole-wheat breadcrumbs before baking until golden brown.

3 TUNA AND AVOCADO POKE
Poke is a Hawaiian dish of very fresh raw chopped fish seasoned with sesame seeds, soy sauce, and scallions. Use sashimi-grade raw tuna and try mixing it with avocado for an extra dimension.

Eating tuna raw makes the most of its nutrients

Tuna and avocado poke ▶

MAXIMIZE THE BENEFITS

CHOOSE FRESH TUNA
Although canned oily fish usually retains omega-3 fatty acids, this isn't the case for tuna, so choose fresh tuna over canned.

EAT REGULARLY IN MODERATION
Experts recommend adults eat at least one portion of oily fish per week to get the benefit, but no more than four portions, because some oily fish may also contain low-level pollutants and mercury that can build up in the body.

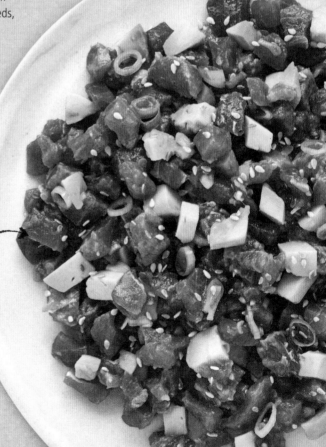

GRILLED SALMON WITH KALE PESTO

Fresh salmon is rich in omega-3 fatty acids, which help keep your heart and brain healthy. Pair it with gut-friendly asparagus, immune-boosting lemons, and a pesto rich in bone-strengthening kale for a nourishing main meal.

Serves 4 **Prep time** 10 minutes **Cook time** 20–30 minutes

INGREDIENTS

1/2 cup **walnut** pieces

1/2 cup young **kale**, washed and deribbed (about1oz/30g)

1 clove **garlic**, crushed

2 tbsp **lemon** juice

6 tbsp olive oil, plus extra for cooking

10 basil leaves

3 tbsp Parmesan cheese, finely grated

salt and freshly ground black pepper

1 bunch **asparagus** (about 14oz/400g), trimmed

1 **lemon,** cut into wedges, to garnish

4 **salmon** fillets, about 5 1/2oz (150g) each, with skin on

SPECIAL EQUIPMENT

blender or small food processor

ridged cast-iron grill pan

METHOD

1 Dry-fry the walnuts in a nonstick frying pan over medium heat for 2–3 minutes, stirring constantly until they are golden brown in places. Transfer onto a clean kitchen towel and rub to remove any excess skin, then let cool.

2 Place the kale, garlic, lemon juice, olive oil, basil, and Parmesan into the blender or food processor. Add the cooled walnuts and season well. Blend to a thick consistency, adding a little more olive oil if needed. Refrigerate until needed.

3 Heat the grill pan over medium-high heat and brush with a little olive oil. Pour a little oil into a shallow dish, then roll the asparagus stalks in the oil and season well. Grill them for 1–2 minutes on each side until they are browned in places. Set aside and keep warm.

4 Wipe the grill pan with paper towels, then brush with oil and grill the lemon wedges for about 30 seconds on each side, until nicely blackened in places. Set aside with the asparagus.

5 Wipe and re-oil the grill pan. Season the salmon fillets well, brush them with oil, and grill over medium-high heat for 2–3 minutes on each side, depending on their thickness and how you like salmon cooked. Grill with the skin side down first to help hold the fish together as it cooks. You may need to cook the salmon in batches to avoid overcrowding the pan.

6 Serve the salmon with the pesto and asparagus, with lemon wedges to garnish. Store leftover pesto in an airtight container in the fridge for up to 5 days.

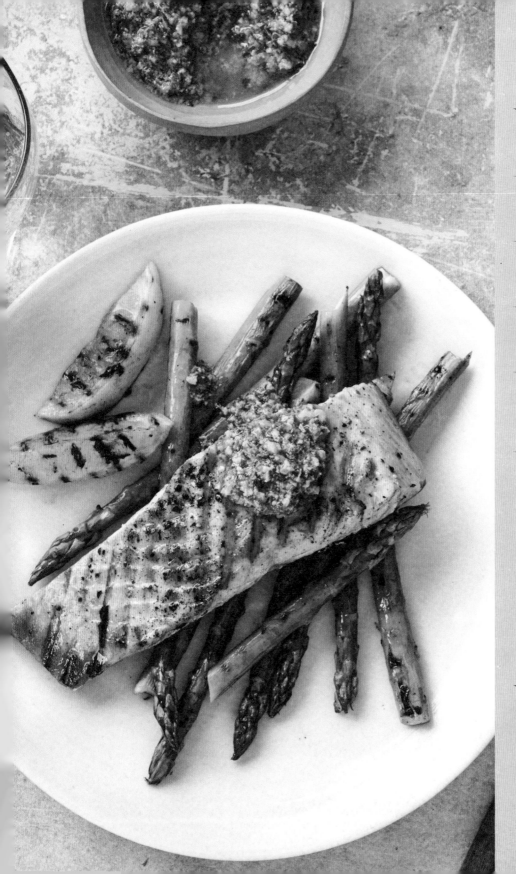

FEATURED SUPERFOODS

WALNUTS
may help boost your
immune system

KALE
helps maintain
healthy bones

GARLIC
may deactivate
cancer-causing agents

LEMON
helps maintain your
immune system

ASPARAGUS
encourages the growth
of **friendly bacteria**
in your gut

SALMON
helps to keep
your **heart** and
brain healthy

Nutrition
per serving

Energy 657cals (2685kj)
Carbohydrate 3g
– of which sugars 3g
Fiber 3.5g
Fat 54g
– of which saturated 9g
Salt 0.2g
Protein 38g
Cholesterol 105mg

POULTRY

Poultry is high in protein and provides B vitamins such as niacin, which helps your body access the energy in foods. Chicken and turkey have superfood status, as they are lower in fat than other poultry meats.

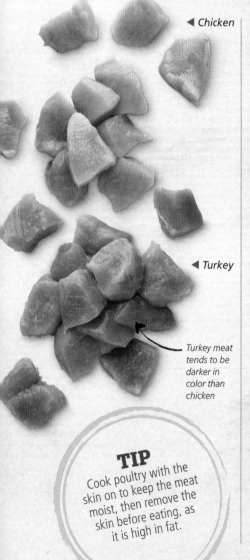

◀ *Chicken*

◀ *Turkey*

Turkey meat tends to be darker in color than chicken

TIP
Cook poultry with the skin on to keep the meat moist, then remove the skin before eating, as it is high in fat.

WHY EAT IT?

DIGESTIVE HEALTH
Chicken and turkey are both high in protein, low in fat, and have a high satiety index (SI), which means that they make you feel fuller for longer. High SI foods tend to be high in protein, fiber, or other nutrients, and are particularly useful for people trying to lose weight.

ANTI-AGING
Rich in protein, poultry protects your body against muscle atrophy, which is particularly important for older people. Sufficient protein intake—about 1¾oz (50g) each day—helps prevent a condition called age-related sarcopenia, which causes loss of strength and mobility, and can increase the risk of falls and fractures.

ENERGY BALANCE
All poultry is a good source of B vitamins, which help to keep your blood healthy and reduce tiredness and fatigue. Vitamin B6 helps your body produce the hormones which influence mood and regulate your body clock.

WHAT'S IN IT?

3½oz (100g) of cooked chicken provides a good source of niacin, phosphorus, potassium, and zinc. Chicken contains slightly more niacin than turkey.

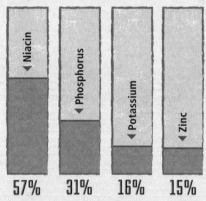

Niacin	Phosphorus	Potassium	Zinc
57%	31%	16%	15%

Percentage of your daily reference intake

Poultry is a good source of **B vitamins**, which help maintain **blood health** and **reduce tiredness** and **fatigue**.

Chicken and **turkey** are high in **protein**, helping your body **build muscle** and protecting against **muscle atrophy** in **older people**. Protein also helps prevent **age-related sarcopenia**, a condition that causes **reduced strength** and **mobility**, increasing the risk of **falls** and **fractures**.

MAXIMIZE THE BENEFITS

CHOOSE DARK MEAT
Darker meat from the thighs and legs of the bird contains higher levels of vitamins and minerals than lighter-colored cuts. However, it also contains more calories and around twice as much fat as breast meat, so consume it in moderate quantities.

COOK IT WITHOUT FAT
The healthiest ways to prepare chicken and turkey use as little added fat as possible during cooking. Try grilling, baking, or poaching poultry for maximum nutritional benefit and minimal fat content.

HOW TO EAT IT

1 ASIAN-STYLE MEATBALLS
Spicy Asian-style meatballs work wonderfully using ground dark chicken meat. Add chile, scallions, cilantro, and lemongrass and pan-fry until golden brown and cooked through. Serve in a salad-stuffed wrap or pita bread.

2 MAKE A STOCK
Cooking chicken or turkey bones for a long time over low heat extracts the maximum flavor and nutrients from the birds. Add onions, carrots, celery, and bay leaves to the pan, top with water, and simmer slowly for a rich, aromatic broth. Use as a base for soups and stews.

3 TURKEY ENDIVE "WRAPS"
Shred cooked turkey and lightly toss it with grated carrots, Greek yogurt, and chopped fresh mint. Pile into individual endive leaves before serving.

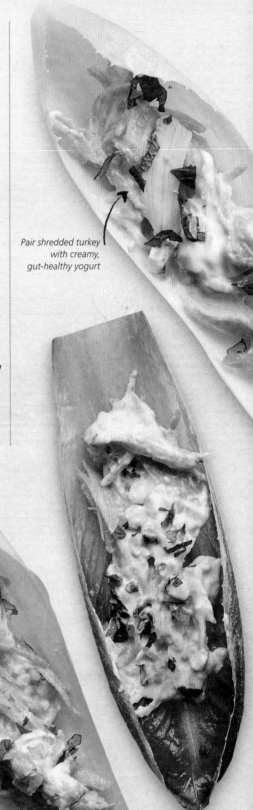

Pair shredded turkey with creamy, gut-healthy yogurt

Endive leaves are rich in fiber

Turkey endive "wraps" ▶

EATING FOR BRAIN HEALTH

Insufficient intake of brain-powering nutrients can cause poor concentration and depression, and increase the risk of Alzheimer's and dementia in later life. Here is an example of a day of eating to boost your brain health.

Antioxidant-rich mint may help protect your brain from damage by free radicals

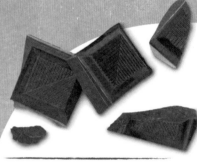

TO DRINK

Drink a large glass of water or mint tea as soon as you wake up to top off your fluid levels after sleep. Studies have shown that drinking a glass of cold water just before completing a brain-taxing task can improve performance by up to 10 percent.

MID-MORNING SNACK

Eat a square of good-quality dark chocolate or a handful of cacao nibs to boost your brain power. Cacao—the principle ingredient in chocolate—contains phytochemicals called flavanoids that are thought to help improve blood flow to the brain. It also contains small quantities of caffeine, which helps you stay alert and focused.

The natural sugars in fruit and honey provide energy for your brain

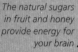

BREAKFAST

Scientists believe that one of the reasons our memory fades with age is because over the course of time our brain cells become damaged by free radicals. Blueberries are packed with antioxidants that help to protect the brain against such damage, so add fresh blueberries to your breakfast bowl for a brain-nourishing start to your day.

Blueberries are rich in brain-protecting antioxidants

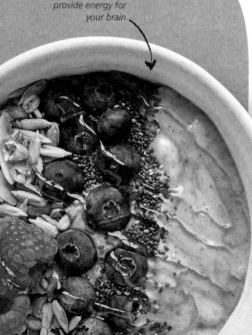

Broccoli may help improve brain function

DINNER

Incorporate oily fish, such as fresh salmon, sardines, mackerel, or tuna, into your evening meal. The omega-3 fatty acids—docosahexaenoic acid (DHA) and eicosapentaenoic acid (EPA)—found in these fish have been shown to improve communication of messages between cells in your brain.

Add mackerel to your dinner for a hit of brain-healthy omega-3 fatty acids

LUNCH

Base your lunch around leafy green vegetables, such as kale or spinach, or cruciferous vegetables, such as broccoli or cabbage. Add proteins such as quinoa and feta or nuts and seeds for a simple salad that nourishes your brain. Researchers at the Brigham and Women's Hospital in Boston found that women who ate at least eight servings of green leafy vegetables and five servings of cruciferous vegetables a week had better memory, verbal ability, and attention levels compared with those who rarely ate them.

AFTERNOON SNACK

Eat a mixed fruit salad to boost your brain and energy levels during the afternoon. Choose vitamin C–rich fruits, such as strawberries, raspberries, orange, papaya, kiwi, and pineapple. People who consume high quantities of vitamin C–rich foods have been found to have better memory recall and attention levels than those who don't.

Avoid low-calorie diets

Low-calorie diets increase reaction times, worsen memory recall, and shorten attention spans.

Base a superfood fruit salad on vitamin C–rich berries

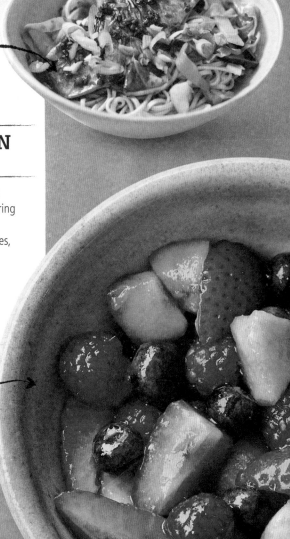

YOGURT

Packed with calcium and "friendly" probiotic bacteria, yogurt helps keep your bones strong and your gut healthy. Yogurt may also help reduce the risk of obesity, diabetes, and some types of cancer.

WHY EAT IT?

BONE STRENGTH

Yogurt is a rich source of calcium, which is vital for forming and maintaining strong, healthy bones. The type of calcium found in yogurt is more easily absorbed than calcium from other food sources. Calcium is particularly important for young people whose bones are still growing—sufficient calcium intake forms bones with strength and rigidity, and reduces the risk of osteoporosis later in life.

DIGESTIVE HEALTH

There are around 400 different strains of bacteria living in your gut, and the live cultures in probiotic yogurt promote "friendly" types of bacteria. Well-balanced gut flora is important both for digestive health and the health of your whole body. The good bacteria in yogurt help reduce the risk of ulcers and inflammatory bowel disease.

DISEASE PREVENTION

Studies have shown that regular consumption of yogurt may help reduce the risk of obesity, diabetes, and some types of cancer. The probiotics in yogurt may be particularly beneficial to those with a compromised immune system.

Yogurt is a rich source of **calcium**, which is vital for forming and maintaining **healthy bones**, particularly during **childhood** and **adolescence**.

WHAT'S IN IT?

A ⅔-cup serving of whole milk yogurt provides a good source of calcium, vitamin B2, potassium, and protein. Yogurt also contains folate.

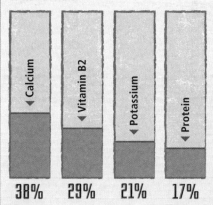

Calcium	Vitamin B2	Potassium	Protein
38%	29%	21%	17%

Percentage of your daily reference intake

Probiotic yogurt is rich in bone-strengthening calcium

MAXIMIZE THE BENEFITS

CHOOSE PROBIOTIC YOGURT
Buy yogurt that is labeled as "probiotic" or "live," as this contains live cultures that boost your gut flora and support your immune system in fending off disease.

GO FOR UNSWEETENED
Yogurt contains natural sugar in the form of lactose, so sugar content can appear high when you look at the nutrition label—always check the ingredients list for added sugar before buying. Fruit yogurt tends to contain a lot of added sugar, so choose natural, unsweetened yogurt and add fresh fruit or fruit purée yourself.

HOW TO PREPARE

To make homemade yogurt, heat 4 cups whole milk to 185°F (85°C), and allow to cool slightly before adding 6 tablespoons live yogurt. Pour into sterilized jars. Allow to ferment in a warm place for 4–6 hours.

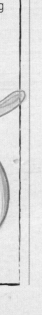

Add live cultures to the milk using store-bought yogurt

HOW TO EAT IT

1 BAKE IT
Baked yogurt makes a refreshing dessert. Simply whisk eggs, Greek yogurt, honey, and a little cornstarch and pour it over fresh blueberries before baking in a low-heat oven until set.

2 IN TZATZIKI
Mix Greek yogurt with grated cucumber, chopped mint, and a little garlic and lemon juice, and serve as a dip, or with broiled meats or fish.

3 YOGURT AND PISTACHIO PANNA COTTA
Greek yogurt can be used in place of cream to make delicate panna cottas. Topped with pistachios and a drizzle of honey or flavored with lavender, they make a light yet satisfying end to a meal.

Yogurt and pistachio panna cotta ▶

The live cultures in yogurt promote **gut-friendly bacteria**, helping to keep your **digestive system** healthy.

TIP
Yogurt made with sheep or goat's milk has a different protein structure from that made with cow's milk, making it easier to digest.

Yogurt can be used as a superfood alternative to cream in many dessert recipes

TURKEY KOFTE

Turkey is high in protein and full of energy-boosting B vitamins, making it the perfect base for these superfood meatballs. Serve with a generous portion of minted citrus yogurt, which supports your immune system and gut health.

Serves 4 **Prep time** 30 minutes, plus chilling **Cook time** 10 minutes

INGREDIENTS

1lb 2oz (500g) ground **turkey**
4 **scallions**, finely chopped
1 tbsp finely chopped **mint**
1 tbsp finely chopped **cilantro**
1 tbsp finely chopped
   flat-leaf **parsley**
2 tbsp finely chopped **pistachios**
1/2 tsp ground coriander
1/2 tsp ground **cumin**
1/4 tsp **cayenne pepper**
salt and freshly ground
   black pepper
olive oil, for cooking

FOR THE CITRUS YOGURT

1 cup Greek-style **yogurt**
zest of 1 large **lemon**
handful of chopped **mint** leaves

FOR THE SALAD

1 tbsp extra-virgin olive oil
1 tbsp Greek-style **yogurt**
2 tbsp **lemon** juice
1 tsp honey
large handfuls of mixed herbs
   such as **mint**, flat-leaf
   parsley, or **cilantro**
3½oz (100g) baby arugula
¼ small red **onion**, finely sliced
seeds from 1 **pomegranate**

METHOD

1 To make the kofte, put all the ingredients into a large bowl, season well, and mix together using your hands until completely combined. Wash your hands, leaving them a little damp, and form 12 equal-sized patties. Place them on a baking sheet lined with wax paper, cover them with plastic wrap, and chill for at least 30 minutes.

2 To make the citrus yogurt, blend all the ingredients together, season well, and chill until needed.

3 To make the salad, whisk the olive oil, yogurt, lemon juice, and honey together in a salad bowl. Season well. Just before serving, toss through the prepared herbs, arugula leaves, sliced onion, and most of the pomegranate seeds.

4 To cook the kofte, heat a little olive oil in a cast-iron frying pan or ridged cast-iron grill pan over medium-high heat. Cook for 4–5 minutes on each side, until the kofte are well browned and springy to the touch.

5 To serve, spread a little citrus yogurt over one side of each plate and place three kofte on top. Put the dressed salad on the other side of the plate and scatter with a few extra pomegranate seeds. Serve immediately.

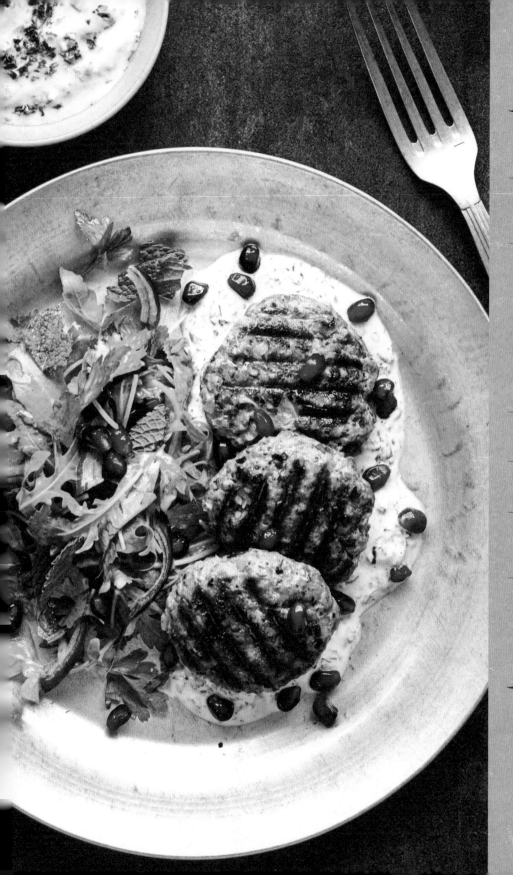

FEATURED SUPERFOODS

TURKEY
helps maintain
muscle strength

ONIONS
encourage the growth
of **gut-friendly bacteria**

HERBS & SPICES
- **Mint** helps boost your immune system
- **Cilantro** helps keep your skin and eyes healthy
- **Parsley** helps maintain healthy bones
- **Cumin** aids digestion
- **Cayenne pepper** may boost your metabolism

PISTACHIOS
help balance **cholesterol**

YOGURT
helps maintain **gut health**

LEMON
helps maintain your
immune system

POMEGRANATE
may help fight **cancer**

Nutrition per serving

Energy 427cals (1738kj)
Carbohydrate 12.5g
– of which sugars 12g
Fiber 3.5g
Fat 17g
– of which saturated 5.5g
Salt 0.4g
Protein 54g
Cholesterol 9g

EGGS

Eggs contain two vital nutrients that are not present in many foods: iodine and vitamin D. Eggs are also rich in tissue-building protein and vitamin B12, which helps your body manufacture blood cells.

WHY EAT IT?

HIGH IN VITAMIN D
Eggs are a good dietary source of vitamin D. Research suggests that people who get enough vitamin D may have a stronger immune system and a reduced risk of multiple sclerosis and certain types of cancer. Vitamin D also helps your body absorb bone-strengthening calcium.

HORMONE BALANCE
Eggs are a useful source of the mineral iodine, which is essential for the manufacture of thyroid hormones. It is also important for the growth of a baby's brain during pregnancy. Nutritional surveys show that many people may not be getting enough iodine in their diet.

HIGH IN PROTEIN
Eggs are an excellent source of protein, which is essential for building tissue in your bones, skin, muscles, and organs. A high-protein diet can reduce the risk of sarcopenia (loss of muscle mass), which is common in older people and can increase the risk of falls and weight gain.

Rich in **vitamin D**, eggs may help **strengthen** your **immune system** and **reduce** the **risk** of **multiple sclerosis** and certain types of **cancer**.

WHAT'S IN IT?

1 large chicken egg provides a good source of vitamins B12 and D, as well as selenium and iodine. Eggs also contain vitamins A and B2, as well as folate.

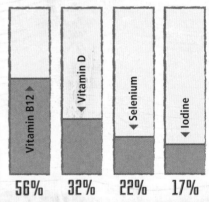

Vitamin B12	Vitamin D	Selenium	Iodine
56%	32%	22%	17%

Percentage of your daily reference intake

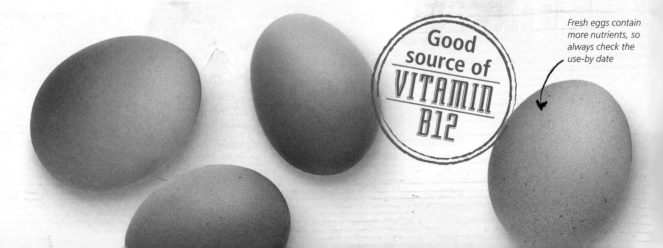

Good source of VITAMIN B12

Fresh eggs contain more nutrients, so always check the use-by date

MAHIMIZE THE BENEFITS

BUY FREE-RANGE AND ORGANIC
Organic, free-range eggs have higher levels of vitamins A and E, and contain less saturated fat than intensively farmed eggs.

TRY DIFFERENT TYPES
All types of egg are rich in protein and B vitamins, but eggs from different birds provide distinct benefits. Chicken eggs contain less cholesterol than other types of egg, and are a good source of vitamins D and B12. Containing more iron and folate than other types of egg, duck eggs help to keep your blood healthy. Goose eggs are similar in nutritional value to chicken eggs, but have a much higher omega-3 fat content, helping protect against heart disease. Quail eggs, though small, are rich in bone-strengthening phosphorus, as well as folate.

HOW TO EAT IT

1 BAKE THEM
Baked eggs make a delicious breakfast or light lunch. Grease a ramekin with olive oil, half-fill with sautéed spinach, season well, then top with an egg and bake until just set.

2 MID-MORNING SNACK
A hard-boiled egg makes a great superfood snack. Rich in protein, it will keep you feeling full until your next meal.

3 FAVA BEAN OMELET
For a lighter version of a Spanish omelet, try substituting the traditional potatoes with freshly shelled fava beans. Sauté the beans with a little garlic in a frying pan. Add beaten egg and chopped fresh herbs, and cook until the top is set and the base is golden brown. Serve warm or at room temperature.

Eggs are a useful source of the mineral **iodine**, which is essential for the manufacture of **thyroid hormones** and the **growth** of a **baby's brain** during **pregnancy**.

TIP
To test an egg for freshness, gently drop it into a glass of cold water. A fresh egg will sink to the bottom of the glass, and a stale egg will float.

Fava bean omelet ▶

Combine a beaten egg with fresh fava beans, which are high in vitamin C and fiber

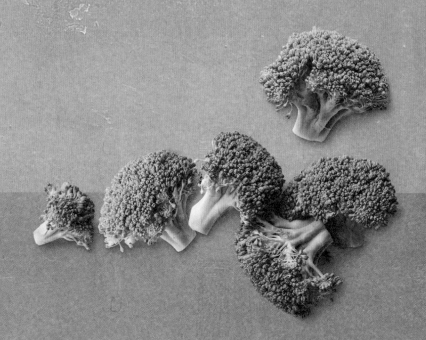

VEGETABLES

CARROTS

An excellent source of vitamin A and the phytochemical beta-carotene, carrots help keep your eyes and bones healthy, and may help protect against several types of cancer.

WHY EAT IT?

ANTI-AGING

Beta-carotene contained in carrots is an antioxidant that helps to protect the skin from free radicals that can accelerate aging. It can also help to improve skin tone and color.

CANCER PREVENTION

Beta-carotene and other carotenoids are known to reduce the risk of certain types of cancer, such as lung cancer. Studies have found that taking beta-carotene supplements does not offer the same positive effects as a diet rich in natural carotenoids.

EYE HEALTH

Beta-carotene may help to maintain eye health—one study found that people with low levels of beta-carotene in their blood were over five times more likely to suffer from cataracts. Carrots also contain lutein and zeaxanthin—carotenoids that help reduce the risk of age-related macular degeneration (AMD).

WHAT'S IN IT?

A ¾-cup serving of raw carrots is an excellent source of vitamin A, and a good source of vitamins K and B1, and the mineral potassium. Carrots also contain vitamins C, B2, and B6, as well as folate, iron, magnesium, phosphorus, zinc, manganese, and fiber.

Vitamin A	Vitamin K	Vitamin B1	Potassium
145%	17%	12%	9%

Percentage of your daily reference intake

Carrot skin is nutritious, so buy organic carrots and eat them unpeeled

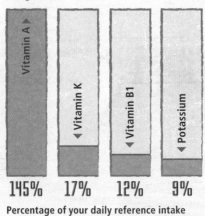

Carrots with bright green tops have been harvested recently, and contain high levels of nutrients

WHERE IS IT FROM?

Modern carrots are descended from wild cultivars that grew—and still grow—in Afghanistan. Wild carrots are purple, red, and yellow in color. Orange carrots were first developed in Holland in the seventeenth century, and are now cultivated in temperate climates all over the world. Although orange carrots are ubiquitous, heritage varieties are gaining popularity. All varieties are at their peak during cooler months.

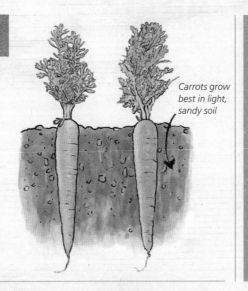

Carrots grow best in light, sandy soil

MAXIMIZE THE BENEFITS

EAT RAW AND COOKED
Although raw carrots provide more vitamin C than cooked carrots, cooking them means the body can absorb 30 percent more beta-carotene.

TOSS WITH OIL
Carotenoids are fat-soluble, so cook carrots with a little fat—for instance, in a stir-fry—to improve their absorption into the body.

HOW TO EAT IT

1 GO RAW
Make a decorative raw salad by using a potato peeler or spiralizer to create ribbons of carrot and zucchini. Toss them with a handful of mint and cilantro, sliced red onion, and an Asian-style salad dressing.

2 ROAST FOR FLAVOR
Roasting root vegetables, such as carrots, really concentrates their flavor. Lightly toss thin baby carrots in olive oil, season to taste, and roast in a hot oven for 30 minutes. Add thyme and garlic cloves for some extra flavor.

3 BAKED ENERGY BITES
Add nutrients and color to some simple, homemade energy bites with carrot. Blend chopped carrots with cooked buckwheat, lightly toasted nuts or seeds, cooked beans, and chopped herbs. Roll the mixture into evenly sized balls and bake in a hot oven for 20 minutes.

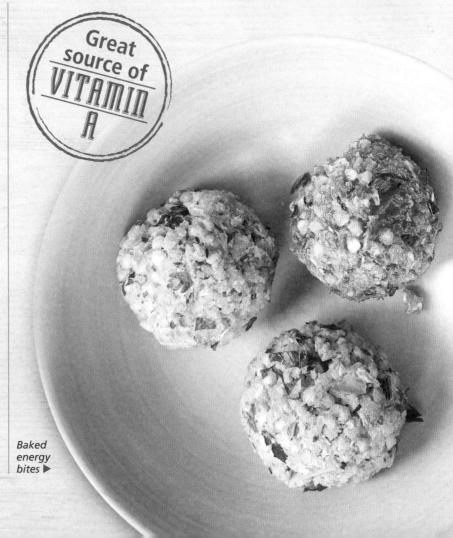

Great source of VITAMIN A

Baked energy bites ▶

SWEET POTATOES

An excellent source of vitamins A and C, sweet potatoes boost your immune system and help keep your skin healthy. They also have a very low glycemic index, providing a steady supply of energy to your body.

WHY EAT IT?

SKIN HEALTH

Sweet potatoes contain high levels of vitamins A and C. Vitamin A helps form and maintain healthy skin, while vitamin C helps your body produce collagen, a protein that is essential for skin health. Sweet potatoes also contain the phytochemical beta-carotene, which helps improve skin color and tone.

IMMUNE BOOST

The high quantities of vitamin C in sweet potatoes help protect the cells that make up the immune system, and support white blood cells in fending off bacteria and viruses.

Eat sweet potatoes with the skin on, as it is high in fiber

ENERGY BALANCE

Sweet potatoes have a low glycemic index (GI), which means that the digestive system converts them into sugar slowly. This helps avoid spikes in blood sugar and provides a steady supply of energy to the body.

Sweet potatoes are an excellent source of **vitamin A**, which helps form and maintain **healthy skin**.

WHAT'S IN IT?

A large, baked sweet potato (6¼oz/180g) provides an excellent source of vitamins A and C, as well as manganese and potassium.

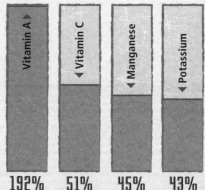

Vitamin A ▶	◀ Vitamin C	◀ Manganese	◀ Potassium
192%	51%	45%	43%

Percentage of your daily reference intake

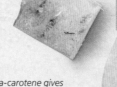

Beta-carotene gives sweet potatoes their vibrant color

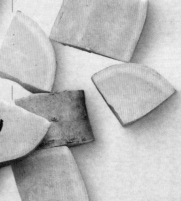

WHERE IS IT FROM?

Native to Central America, sweet potatoes are now widely cultivated in warm, temperate regions across the world, including the tropics. In spite of their name, they are not related to ordinary potatoes, but are part of the *Convolvulaceae* family. They come in a range of colors, from white to orange, but orange-fleshed varieties are the most popular.

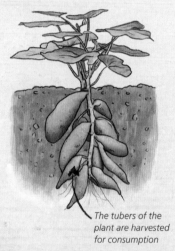

The tubers of the plant are harvested for consumption

MAXIMIZE THE BENEFITS

EAT WITH A LITTLE FAT
Combine sweet potatoes with a little fat such as avocado, nuts, or olive oil—this helps your body absorb the nutrients.

CHOOSE ORANGE
Choose varieties of sweet potato that have vibrant orange flesh, as these contain more beta-carotene. Beta-carotene is a phytochemical that supports healthy skin.

HOW TO EAT IT

1 ROAST THEM
Roast sweet potatoes in an Asian-inspired marinade. Blend a little maple syrup with some reduced-sodium soy sauce. Add chunks of sweet potatoes, sprinkle with sesame seeds, and roast in a hot oven for about 30 minutes.

2 IN A WRAP
Roasted sweet potatoes make a satisfying filling in a wrap with hummus and baby spinach.

3 SWEET POTATO SOUP
Use leftover baked sweet potatoes as a base for a quick, satisfying soup. Cook onion, garlic, and ginger, then add diced sweet potatoes and vegetable stock. Cook until soft, then blend and top with grated nutmeg or toasted pumpkin seeds.

Sweet potato soup ▶

Sweet potatoes contain **high levels** of **vitamin C**, which is required for a **strong** and **healthy immune system**.

TIP
Store sweet potatoes at cool room temperature, away from sunlight. Avoid storing them in the fridge, as this causes them to lose flavor.

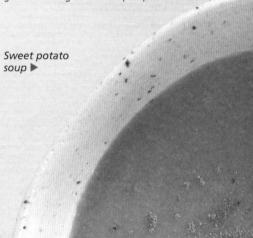

SWEET POTATO & BLACK BEAN QUESADILLAS

Beta-carotene-rich sweet potatoes support your immune system and keep your skin healthy. In these vegetarian quesadillas, they're paired with beans and avocado, both of which keep your heart healthy and balance cholesterol.

Serves 4 **Prep time** 35 minutes **Cook time** 8–12 minutes

INGREDIENTS

4 tbsp olive oil, plus extra for cooking

2 large **sweet potatoes**, peeled and finely diced, about 1lb 2oz (500g) total weight

½ small red **onion**, finely diced

1 mild green chile, seeded and very finely chopped

1 large beefsteak **tomato**, peeled, seeded, and finely chopped

1 (14oz; 400g) can **black beans**, drained and rinsed

large handful of fresh **cilantro** leaves, roughly chopped

2½oz (75g) grated cheese, such as Cheddar or red Leicester

1 scant tsp smoked paprika

8 (8in; 20cm) soft corn or flour tortillas

FOR THE AVOCADO SALSA

2 ripe **avocados**, finely chopped

4 **scallions**, finely chopped

1 tbsp olive oil

juice of 1 lime

2 tbsp finely chopped **cilantro**

METHOD

1 To make the avocado salsa, simply mix all the ingredients together, season well, and refrigerate until needed.

2 To make the quesadilla filling, heat 3 tablespoons of the olive oil in a large, nonstick frying pan. Cook the sweet potatoes over medium-high heat for 10 minutes, stirring occasionally, until softened and golden brown in places. Add the remaining oil, onion, and chile, and cook for another 5 minutes.

3 Add the chopped tomato and cook for a final 5 minutes, stirring frequently, until the tomato starts to break down. Remove from the heat.

4 Add the drained black beans and use a potato masher to gently crush the mixture. Add the chopped cilantro, grated cheese, and smoked paprika, and season well. Mix well to combine.

5 Preheat the oven to 250°F (130°C). Heat a little oil in a large, clean nonstick frying pan. Meanwhile, spread one quarter of the mixture over one tortilla and top with a second, pressing down to sandwich them together. Cook over medium heat for 2–3 minutes on each side, turning once carefully, until golden brown all over. Place on a baking sheet and keep warm in the oven while you cook the rest of the quesadillas.

6 To serve, cut the quesadillas into quarters and serve with a little of the avocado salsa alongside.

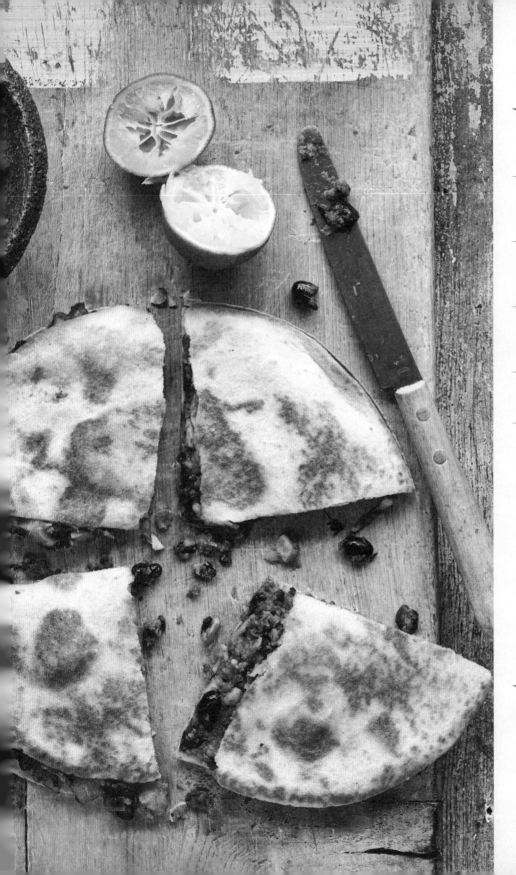

FEATURED SUPERFOODS

SWEET POTATOES
help maintain your
immune system

ONIONS
encourage the growth
of **gut-friendly bacteria**

TOMATOES
may reduce the risk of
heart-related diseases

BLACK BEANS
may help reduce **high
cholesterol** levels

CILANTRO
supports **eye health**

AVOCADOS
help maintain healthy
cholesterol levels and
protect the **heart**

Nutrition
per serving

Energy 881cals (3558kj)
Carbohydrate 90g
– of which sugars 14g
Fiber 18g
Fat 45g
– of which saturated 12g
Salt 1.8g
Protein 20g
Cholesterol 18g

BEETS

Beets contain phytochemicals called nitrates that help to keep your blood and heart healthy and may help slow the progression of dementia. They are also a rich source of folate, which helps your body produce red blood cells.

WHY EAT IT?

BLOOD HEALTH
Beets are a good source of nitrates, which are converted into nitric oxide in your body. Nitric oxide helps relax and dilate blood vessels, helping reduce high blood pressure. Beets are also rich in folate, a B vitamin that helps your body produce hemoglobin, the protein in red blood cells that carries oxygen.

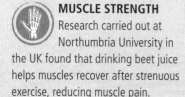

MUSCLE STRENGTH
Research carried out at Northumbria University in the UK found that drinking beet juice helps muscles recover after strenuous exercise, reducing muscle pain.

BRAIN POWER
Studies show that the nitrates found in beets may help slow the progression of dementia by helping to improve blood flow to your brain.

WHAT'S IN IT?

A ¾-cup serving of raw beets is a good source of folate, manganese, potassium, and iron. Beets also contain vitamins A, B1, B2, B6, C, and niacin, as well as calcium, magnesium, zinc, copper, and selenium.

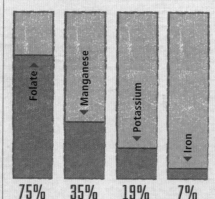

Folate ►	◄ Manganese	◄ Potassium	◄ Iron
75%	35%	19%	7%

Percentage of your daily reference intake

Drinking **beet juice** may help reduce **muscle pain** and **soreness** after **strenuous exercise**.

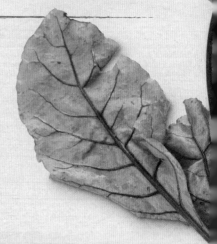

MAXIMIZE THE BENEFITS

EAT IT RAW OR LIGHTLY COOKED
Raw beets contain maximum nitrate levels. Boiling beets causes the nitrates to leach out into the water, so boil it only until just ready and use the cooking water as stock for soup or gravy.

CHOOSE DIFFERENT VARIETIES
The most common, dark purple variety of beets is rich in betacyanin, a pigment that may help protect against cancer. Beets with bright yellow flesh contain pigments called betaxanthins, which may help boost immunity.

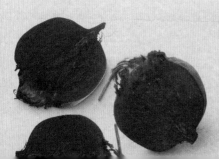

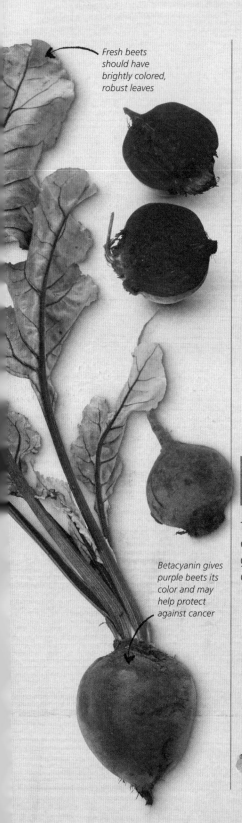

Fresh beets should have brightly colored, robust leaves

Beet and barley risotto ▶

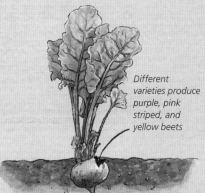

TIP
Cook beets with the skin on to preserve nutrients, then eat with the skin on or peel when cooled.

Betacyanin gives purple beets its color and may help protect against cancer

WHERE IS IT FROM?

The edible roots of the beet plant have been eaten for thousands of years. The modern garden beet was developed in the sixteenth century and grows in temperate climates.

Different varieties produce purple, pink striped, and yellow beets

HOW TO EAT IT

1 BEET AND BARLEY RISOTTO
Puréed beets give a rich, vibrant color to risottos. Prepare a superfood risotto by lightly toasting barley, then using it as a base for risotto, mixing in cooked, puréed beets toward the end.

2 ADD TO BROWNIES
The earthy flavor of beets pair extremely well with rich, dark cacao. Try the ultimate superfood brownies that mix lightly cooked and puréed beets with cacao powder and maple syrup into flour and eggs.

3 RAW JUICE
Extract all the goodness from raw beets by juicing them. Use well-scrubbed baby beets, and juice with the skins on. The dark red color makes a good base for any kind of breakfast juice.

BUTTERNUT SQUASH

All varieties of squash are nutritious, but butternut squash is a superfood because it contains high levels of carotenoids, which help combat cancer and support skin health.

WHY EAT IT?

CANCER PREVENTION
Rich in carotenoid compounds including beta-carotene, butternut squash helps protect against certain types of cancer.

IMMUNE BOOST
Butternut squash is a useful source of vitamin C, which protects your immune system and boosts the action of white blood cells.

SKIN HEALTH
Packed with beta-carotene and vitamin A, butternut squash helps your body renew skin cells. Beta-carotene has also been shown to improve skin tone and appearance, making your skin look healthier.

Cancer-fighting carotenoids give butternut squash its bright color

WHAT'S IN IT?

A ½-cup serving of baked butternut squash provides a good source of vitamins A and C, as well as potassium and folate.

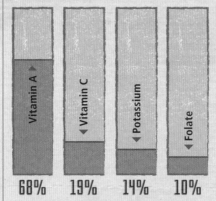

Vitamin A	Vitamin C	Potassium	Folate
68%	19%	14%	10%

Percentage of your daily reference intake

HOW TO EAT IT

1 ROASTED SQUASH
The easiest way to prepare a butternut squash is to halve it, seed it, and roast it in a hot oven until soft.

2 VEGETARIAN LASAGNA
Very thinly slice butternut squash, and use it as a wheat-free alternative to lasagna sheets in a shiitake mushroom and spinach lasagna.

3 DAIRY-FREE SAUCE
Puréed butternut squash makes a colorful, dairy-free sauce for pasta—combine it with a little almond milk and season with salt, pepper, and nutmeg.

WHERE IS IT FROM?

Butternut squash is a cold-season squash in the gourd family. Squashes were first cultivated in the Americas over 7,000 years ago.

Butternut squashes are harvested in the fall

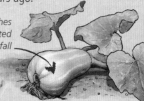

FENNEL

Traditionally used to aid digestion, fennel contains phytochemicals that soothe your stomach. Fennel may also help reduce high blood pressure.

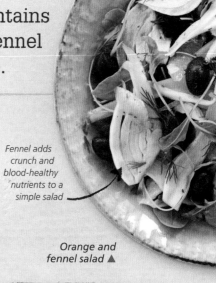

WHY EAT IT?

DIGESTIVE HEALTH
Fennel contains a phytochemical called anethole, which is believed to aid digestion by stimulating digestive juices. Drinking fennel tea may help relieve flatulence and bloating.

BLOOD HEALTH
A good source of potassium and folate, fennel supports blood health by helping regulate blood pressure and manufacture red blood cells. Fennel also contains nitrates that relax and dilate your blood vessels, helping to reduce high blood pressure.

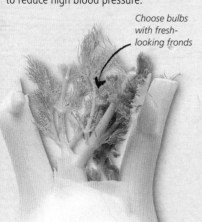

Choose bulbs with fresh-looking fronds

WHAT'S IN IT?

A 1-cup serving of fennel provides a good source of potassium, folate, vitamin C, and fiber.

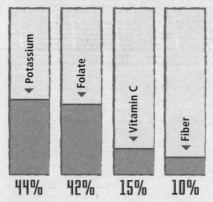

Potassium	Folate	Vitamin C	Fiber
44%	**42%**	**15%**	**10%**

Percentage of your daily reference intake

WHERE IS IT FROM?

The fennel bulb is the swollen base of the stem of the fennel plant, which grows in temperate climates.

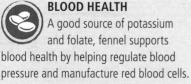

Fennel plants grow to about 3ft (1m) tall

Fennel adds crunch and blood-healthy nutrients to a simple salad

Orange and fennel salad ▲

HOW TO EAT IT

1 ORANGE AND FENNEL SALAD
Combine thinly sliced fennel bulb with fresh orange segments, salad leaves, and olives, and dress with a little olive oil—the orange brings its own acidity.

2 ROAST IT
Roasting fennel enhances its natural aniseed flavor. Toss in a little olive oil and roast in a medium oven for 20–30 minutes. Combine with cooked quinoa and pomegranate seeds for a light meal.

3 BAKE IT
Baked fennel makes an excellent side dish for fish or chicken. Thickly slice, season well, and top with a little olive oil and Parmesan cheese before baking until soft and golden brown on top.

ROASTED SQUASH & BARLEY SALAD

This salad is based on whole-grain pearl barley, which is an excellent source of gut-friendly fiber and helps lower bad cholesterol. Squash provides carotenoid compounds that may help protect against cancer.

Serves 4   **Prep time** 20 minutes, plus overnight soaking   **Cook time** 30 minutes, plus cooling

INGREDIENTS

1¼ cups pearl **barley**, soaked overnight in cold water

juice of 2 **lemons**, plus extra, to taste

2 tbsp extra-virgin olive oil, plus extra for roasting

salt and freshly ground black pepper

1 small acorn or **butternut squash**, about 1lb 5oz (600g) total weight

1 red **onion**, peeled

2 large handfuls of **kale**, washed, deribbed, and finely shredded

2 tbsp coarsely chopped flat-leaf **parsley**

2 tbsp **pumpkin seeds**

1 cup feta cheese, crumbled

METHOD

1 Preheat the oven to 425°F (220°C). Drain and rinse the soaked barley. Put it in a large saucepan of water and bring to a boil. Reduce to a low simmer and cook for 30 minutes, until it is just soft but still has a bite to it.

2 Drain the cooked barley and place it in a heatproof bowl. Dress the barley with the lemon juice and 2 tablespoons of olive oil while it is still warm, and season well. Let it cool while you prepare the rest of the salad.

3 Trim both ends of the squash and cut it into 16 wedges—do not peel it, as the skin contains beneficial fiber and tastes delicious. Seed the squash pieces, toss in a little olive oil, and spread out in a single layer on a large baking sheet. Season well and cook in the top of the oven for 20–25 minutes, turning them halfway through the cooking time, so that they brown on both sides. Remove from the oven and let cool.

4 Meanwhile, cut the red onion into 8 wedges and toss in a little olive oil. Put the wedges in a single layer on another baking sheet, season well, and cook in the oven for 20 minutes, turning them halfway through so they are browned on both sides and a little charred at the edges. Remove from the oven and let cool.

5 To assemble the salad, first check the seasoning of the cooled barley and add extra lemon, olive oil, and salt and pepper if needed. Place the kale in a bowl, drizzle with a little olive oil and salt, and massage it with your hands for a couple of minutes to soften the leaves. Toss the barley with the prepared kale, onion, parsley, pumpkin seeds, and three-quarters of the crumbled feta.

6 Transfer the salad to a large serving bowl and place the wedges of roasted squash in and around the barley. Sprinkle the reserved feta on top and serve.

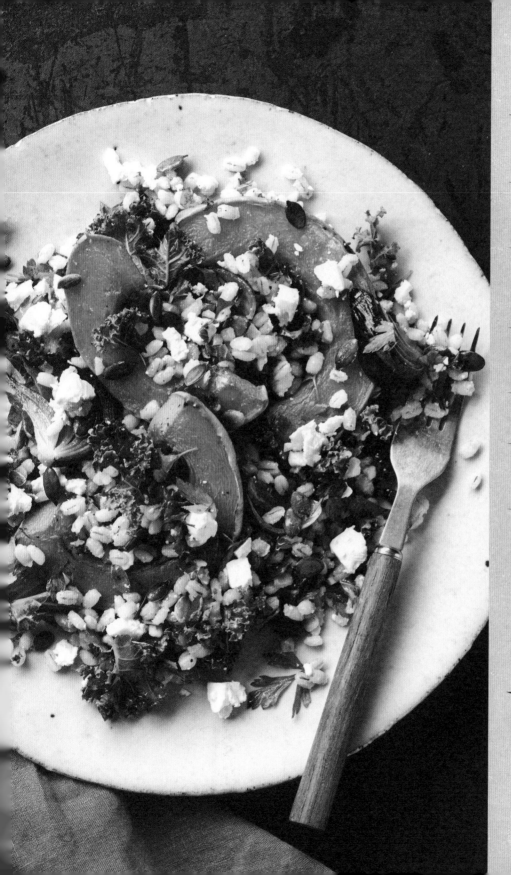

FEATURED SUPERFOODS

BARLEY
helps reduce
bad cholesterol

LEMON
helps maintain your
immune system

BUTTERNUT SQUASH
may help protect
against certain types
of **cancer**

ONIONS
encourage the growth
of **gut-friendly bacteria**

KALE
supports **skin health**

PARSLEY
helps maintain
healthy bones

PUMPKIN SEEDS
are good for
skin health

Nutrition per serving

Energy	535cals (2171kj)
Carbohydrate	67g
– of which sugars	10g
Fiber	6g
Fat	21g
– of which saturated	7g
Salt	1g
Protein	16g
Cholesterol	26g

ONIONS

This humble vegetable is packed with vitamins, minerals, and phytochemicals. Regular consumption of onions can help boost digestive health, reduce the risk of developing heart disease, and prevent several types of cancer.

WHY EAT IT?

DIGESTIVE HEALTH
Onions contain a type of fiber that acts as a probiotic, encouraging the growth of friendly bacteria in the bowel.

HEART HEALTH
Research suggests that onions may help reduce high blood pressure—studies have found that onions may help to thin the blood, helping keep arteries clear of blockages. Quercetin, a phytochemical found in onions, is believed to help reduce the risk of heart disease by helping to prevent bad cholesterol from being deposited in the coronary arteries.

CANCER PREVENTION
The phytochemical quercetin, which is contained in onions, has been shown to inhibit the growth of cancer cells. Some studies show that people who eat onions regularly have a lower risk of developing cancers of the esophagus, colon, breast, ovaries, and kidneys.

WHAT'S IN IT?

¾ cup of raw onion provides a useful source of folate, vitamins B1 and B6, and potassium. Onions also contain vitamins B2, C, and E, as well as fiber, niacin, magnesium, and copper.

Folate	Vitamin B1	Vitamin B6	Potassium
11%	10%	7%	7%

Percentage of your daily reference intake

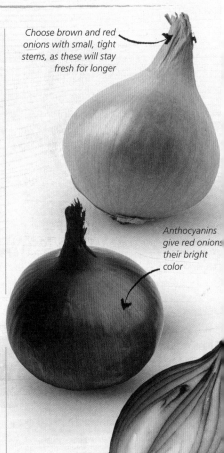

Choose brown and red onions with small, tight stems, as these will stay fresh for longer

Anthocyanins give red onions their bright color

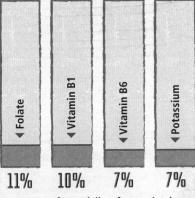

Scallions are onions that are harvested before the bulb grows

Onions contain high levels of **quercetin**, a **phytochemical** that has been found to **reduce** the risk of **heart disease** by preventing **bad cholesterol** from forming in your arteries. Quercetin may also **inhibit** the growth of **cancer cells**.

HOW TO EAT IT

1 QUICK PICKLES
For an almost instant garnish for tacos or burgers, slice a red onion thinly and marinate for 30 minutes in rice wine vinegar sweetened with a little honey, salt, and pepper.

2 IN EGG-FRIED RICE
For a simple Asian-inspired dinner, stir-fry thinly sliced scallions with cooked brown rice, spring vegetables, egg, and a dash of soy sauce.

3 RED ONION AND ORANGE SALAD
Pair mild red onions with sweet, sharp orange slices for a simple side salad. Toss finely sliced red onion with plump green olives and slices of orange, dress with olive oil and fresh lemon juice, and finish with chopped cilantro and a sprinkle of paprika.

TIP
To make nutrient-rich raw onions more mild and easier to eat, dress them with vinegar or serve them with acidic fruits.

MAXIMIZE THE BENEFITS

TRY RED ONIONS
Onions come in many shapes, sizes, and colors, but there is very little difference in the levels of vitamins and minerals between the varieties. However, red onions contain the highest levels of quercetin, a phytochemical that helps reduce bad cholesterol and protect against cancer. Red onions are also richer in anthocyanins—antioxidant phytochemicals that may help keep your heart healthy.

▼ *Red onion and orange salad*

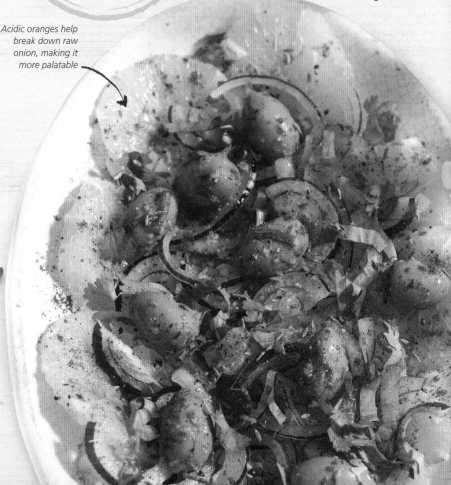

Acidic oranges help break down raw onion, making it more palatable

GARLIC

It is only recently that scientists have begun to identify the components responsible for garlic's myriad health benefits. Rich in phytochemicals and potassium, garlic helps boost your immune system, fight cancer, and protect your heart.

WHY EAT IT?

✓ CANCER PREVENTION
Garlic contains a number of beneficial phytochemicals, including a group of compounds called allyl sulfides that can deactivate cancer-causing agents. Studies show a link between regular garlic consumption and reduced risk of some types of cancer, particularly stomach, bowel, and breast cancer.

Use fresh garlic cloves that are sealed, without green sprouts

IMMUNE BOOST
Scientists believe that garlic can help to strengthen the immune system by stimulating the production of cells that fight bacteria and viruses.

♥ HEART HEALTH
A recent report collated the results of 26 different studies that researched the effects of garlic on blood fats. The report confirmed that regular consumption of garlic can help reduce bad, low-density lipoprotein (LPL) cholesterol and increase good, high-density lipoprotein (HDL) cholesterol. Other studies suggest that garlic can protect the heart by helping to reduce high blood pressure.

Roast garlic bulbs whole in their skins to help preserve antioxidants

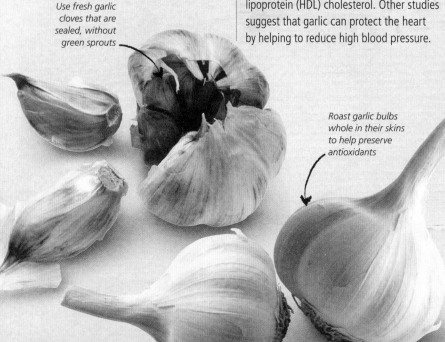

WHAT'S IN IT?

¾ cup of raw garlic provides a good source of potassium, phosphorus, vitamin C, and manganese. Garlic also contains vitamins B1 and B2, as well as selenium.

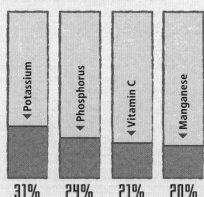

▼Potassium	▼Phosphorus	▼Vitamin C	▼Manganese
31%	24%	21%	20%

Percentage of your daily reference intake

Regular **garlic consumption** has been shown to **reduce bad cholesterol** and **increase good cholesterol**.

WHERE IS IT FROM?

Native to Central Asia, garlic is one of the oldest cultivated food plants. It is a member of the onion family and can be grown throughout the year in mild climates around the world. Garlic is usually harvested when the bulb is round and mature, and then dried before use.

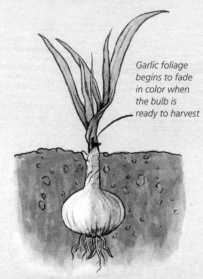

Garlic foliage begins to fade in color when the bulb is ready to harvest

MAXIMIZE THE BENEFITS

LET IT STAND
Crush or chop garlic and allow it to stand for 10–15 minutes before using in recipes. Letting the garlic stand triggers an enzyme reaction that boosts levels of a compound called allicin, which is believed to be responsible for many health benefits.

EAT IT RAW
Cooking garlic reduces allicin levels, so for maximum health benefits, eat it raw.

HOW TO EAT IT

1 ROAST IT WHOLE
Roasted garlic is a fragrant delight. Cut the very top of the bulb off to expose all the cloves, then drizzle with olive oil, season, and bake in a hot oven until caramelized and soft to the touch.

2 CHILLED SOUP
The Spanish soup *ajo blanco* is made by blending breadcrumbs with ground almonds, garlic, olive oil, and water. Chill the mixture and then serve it with a splash of red wine vinegar.

3 GARLIC AND SHRIMP ZUCCHINI "SPAGHETTI"
Spiralized zucchini makes a nutrient-rich alternative to pasta or noodles. To counteract their mild flavor, load them with plenty of chile and garlic, sautéed in a little olive oil until fragrant.

Garlic and shrimp zucchini "spaghetti" ▶

Studies have shown that **eating garlic regularly** leads to a **reduced risk** of developing some types of **cancer**, particularly **stomach**, **bowel**, and **breast cancers**.

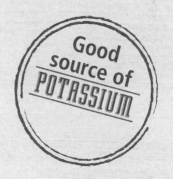

Good source of POTASSIUM

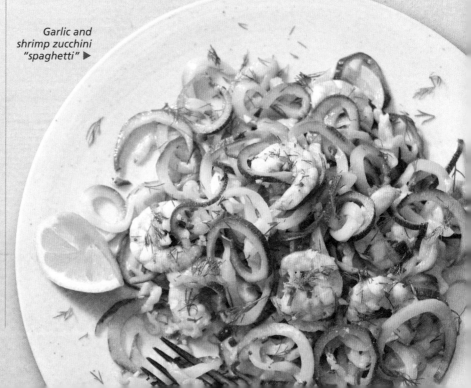

EATING FOR IMMUNITY

The immune system plays a fundamental role in helping to keep you healthy by protecting against infections such as colds and flu, as well as more serious illnesses such as cancer. Here is an example of a day of eating to boost your immune system, which may help increase your resistance to infection and disease.

TO DRINK

Drink a glass of freshly squeezed orange juice to boost your levels of immune-boosting vitamin C. For a more substantial drink, blend yourself a banana and yogurt smoothie—this will encourage the development of healthy bacteria in your gut, helping your body stay healthy and fend off illness.

The vitamin C in oranges helps combat viruses

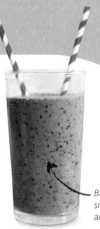

Base your breakfast smoothie on banana and yogurt

MID-MORNING SNACK

Grab an orange for your morning snack. Oranges are packed with vitamin C, which increases the production of infection-fighting white blood cells. Vitamin C also boosts levels of interferon, an antibody that coats the surface of cells, preventing the entry of viruses.

Eating whole-grain cereals reduces the chance of developing colds and flu

BREAKFAST

Eat a simple bowl of yogurt, oats, and fresh fruit for breakfast. Studies show that people who eat whole-grain cereals at breakfast are less likely to suffer from colds and flu. Eating just one small container of yogurt each day can reduce the risk of catching a cold by up to 25 percent.

Good bacteria in yogurt boost your immune system

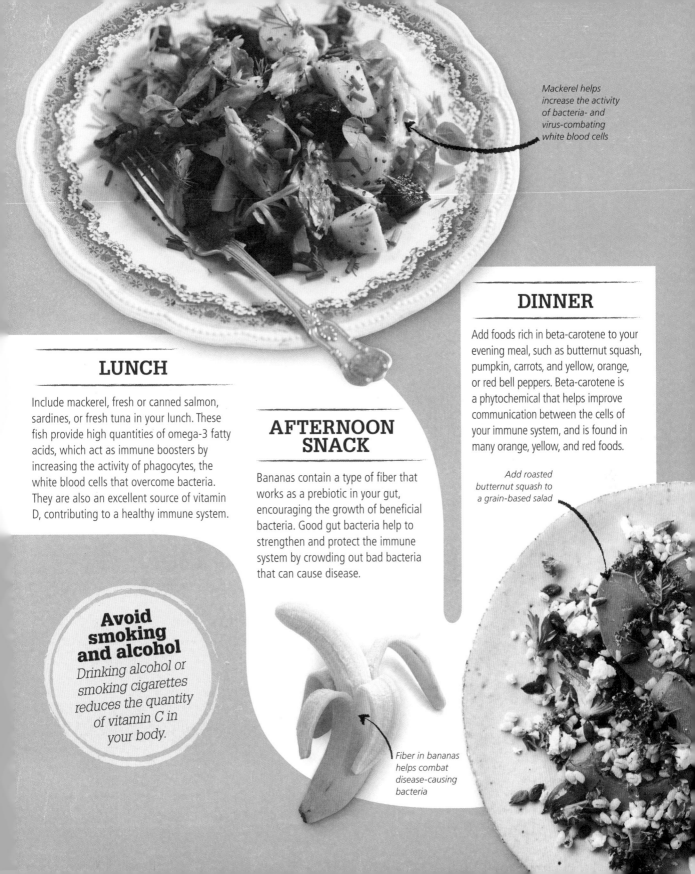

Mackerel helps increase the activity of bacteria- and virus-combating white blood cells

LUNCH

Include mackerel, fresh or canned salmon, sardines, or fresh tuna in your lunch. These fish provide high quantities of omega-3 fatty acids, which act as immune boosters by increasing the activity of phagocytes, the white blood cells that overcome bacteria. They are also an excellent source of vitamin D, contributing to a healthy immune system.

AFTERNOON SNACK

Bananas contain a type of fiber that works as a prebiotic in your gut, encouraging the growth of beneficial bacteria. Good gut bacteria help to strengthen and protect the immune system by crowding out bad bacteria that can cause disease.

DINNER

Add foods rich in beta-carotene to your evening meal, such as butternut squash, pumpkin, carrots, and yellow, orange, or red bell peppers. Beta-carotene is a phytochemical that helps improve communication between the cells of your immune system, and is found in many orange, yellow, and red foods.

Add roasted butternut squash to a grain-based salad

Avoid smoking and alcohol
Drinking alcohol or smoking cigarettes reduces the quantity of vitamin C in your body.

Fiber in bananas helps combat disease-causing bacteria

WATERCRESS

By weight, watercress contains more vitamin C than oranges, and it is also rich in bone-strengthening vitamin K. Phytochemicals in watercress help combat cancer and protect your eyes.

WHY EAT IT?

CANCER PREVENTION
Watercress contains several phytochemicals that are believed to help reduce the risk of cancer. One is phenylethyl isothiocyanate (PEITC), thought to suppress the development of breast cancer cells by starving the growing tumor of blood and oxygen.

BONE STRENGTH
Vitamin K, which is plentiful in watercress, may help prevent osteoporosis and osteoarthritis. Antibiotics can cause a deficiency in vitamin K, so eat watercress to boost levels of this vitamin.

EYE HEALTH
The phytochemicals lutein and zeaxanthin found in watercress help protect the lens and retina of the eye from damage by free radicals and help to delay age-related macular degeneration (AMD). The vitamin C in watercress helps reduce the risk of cataracts.

WHAT'S IN IT?

3½oz (100g) of watercress provides an excellent source of vitamins K, C, and A, as well as folate. Watercress also contains vitamins B1, B2, B6, and E, as well as iron.

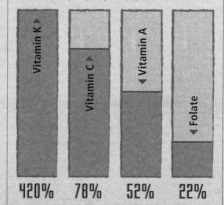

Vitamin K	Vitamin C	Vitamin A	Folate
420%	78%	52%	22%

Percentage of your daily reference intake

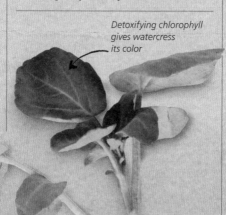

Detoxifying chlorophyll gives watercress its color

HOW TO EAT IT

1 WATERCRESS SALAD
The sharp taste of watercress pairs well with sweet ingredients. Toss watercress with slices of roasted beet or orange segments for a bright-tasting salad.

2 GREEN SMOOTHIE
Add a handful of watercress to the more usual green smoothie ingredients such as spinach and kale for an added boost of vitamin K and phytochemicals.

3 BLEND A DIP
Blend fresh watercress with Greek yogurt, lemon zest, and salt and pepper for an almost instant dip for a plate of freshly chopped raw vegetables.

WHERE IS IT FROM?

A Eurasian native, watercress has spread around the world. It is an aquatic perennial herb, favoring running water.

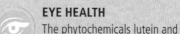

Watercress is grown in springwater over gravel

SPINACH

Packed with folate, vitamin C, and potassium, spinach helps keep your blood, immune system, and eyes healthy.

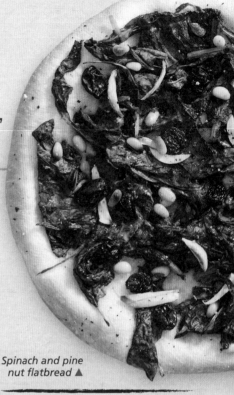

Spinach and pine nut flatbread ▲

WHY EAT IT?

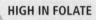

BLOOD HEALTH
Spinach is a good source of potassium, which helps lower high blood pressure by counteracting the negative effects of sodium.

HIGH IN FOLATE
Spinach is an excellent source of folate, which is needed for the production of red blood cells and release of energy from food. Folate is also important in pregnancy to help prevent neural tube defects like spina bifida. Some studies suggest it may offer protection against cancers of the breast and colon.

EYE HEALTH
The phytochemicals lutein and zeaxanthin in spinach can help protect the eyes from damage by free radicals.

WHAT'S IN IT?

3½oz (100g) of baby spinach provides a good source of folate, vitamin C, potassium, and vitamin A. Spinach also contains vitamins B1, B2, and B6, as well as iron.

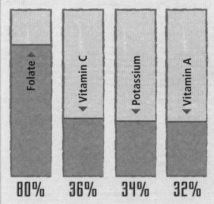

Folate ▶	◀ Vitamin C	◀ Potassium	◀ Vitamin A
80%	36%	34%	32%

Percentage of your daily reference intake

WHERE IS IT FROM?

Native to Iran, spinach is grown in temperate zones worldwide. It is harvested from spring until fall.

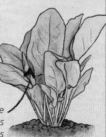

Different varieties produce leaves of varying sizes and textures

HOW TO EAT IT

1 SPINACH AND PINE NUT FLATBREAD
To make this delicious alternative to pizza, wilt spinach in olive oil and garlic, then squeeze it dry, arrange on a flatbread, and top with pine nuts and roasted garlic.

2 SIMPLE SOUP
Cook onions and garlic before adding frozen spinach and stock and cooking for 10 minutes. Purée it with a spoonful of Greek yogurt, until smooth.

3 IN A SALAD
Raw baby spinach leaves are milder than more mature spinach. Dress with a vibrant vinaigrette and garnish with toasted nuts and seeds.

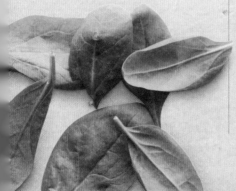

KALE

Low in calories and high in vitamins K, C, A, and the B vitamin folate, kale supports your eyesight, bones, and circulation, making it a key superfood at any stage of life. Kale is also a rich source of antioxidant phytochemicals.

WHY EAT IT?

EYE HEALTH
Kale is rich in a phytochemical called lutein, an antioxidant that protects eyes from damage from sunlight. Studies show that eating a diet rich in lutein can reduce the risk of age-related macular degeneration (AMD), which is the most common cause of loss of vision in older people. It is also rich in vitamin A, which is important for healthy eyes.

BONE STRENGTH
A good source of calcium, kale helps maintain healthy bones—making it an especially useful superfood for people who don't eat dairy. It also contains vitamin K, which works with calcium to keep the bones strong.

Kale leaves are rich in gut-friendly fiber

Curly kale ▶

BLOOD HEALTH
Kale is rich in folate (one of the B vitamins) and iron, both of which are needed for the production of red blood cells. Folate is also important for women who are planning to become pregnant, because it helps to protect against birth defects.

Kale is a good source of **calcium**, especially important for people who follow a **dairy-free diet**.

WHAT'S IN IT?

1 cup of raw kale provides an excellent source of vitamins K, C, A, and folate, as well as calcium, iron, and B vitamins.

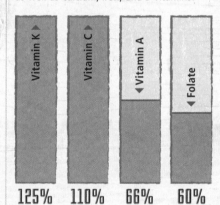

Vitamin K	Vitamin C	Vitamin A	Folate
125%	110%	66%	60%

Percentage of your daily reference intake

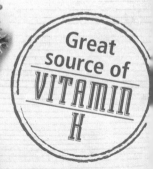

Great source of VITAMIN K

Kale is rich in a **phytochemical** called **lutein**. Lutein can help **reduce** the risk of age-related **macular degeneration**, which is the most common cause of **loss of vision** in older people.

MAXIMIZE THE BENEFITS

BUY ORGANIC
Organic kale holds twice as many nutrients as nonorganic kale.

EAT RAW AND COOKED
Raw kale contains more vitamin C and B vitamins than cooked kale, but cooking it boosts levels of other nutrients, including iron, so enjoy it both raw and cooked.

TOSS WITH OIL
Adding fat to kale when you cook it or serve it helps the body absorb its nutrients.

WHERE IS IT FROM?

Kale is descended from the wild cabbages of southern Europe. Modern varieties are hardy, and are now grown around the world in cold to temperate climates. Frosts sweeten up its leaves, so kale is usually harvested in autumn and winter. The curly-leaved cultivar is the most popular variety in Europe and North America, and the dark-leaved lacinato kale, or cavolo nero, is widely used in Tuscan cooking.

Different varieties produce blue-green, light green, red, or purple leaves

▲ *Kale and root vegetable soup*

HOW TO EAT IT

1 KALE AND ROOT VEGETABLE SOUP
Kale makes a simple yet wholesome addition to soups and stews. Coarsely chop it and blend into a flavorful root vegetable soup for added color, flavor, and nutrients.

2 KALE CHIPS
To make the ultimate healthy snack, wash and dry kale well, de-rib and tear into 1in (3cm) pieces, rub with a little olive oil, and bake in a single layer in a preheated 275°F (140°C) oven for 20 minutes, turning occasionally. Sprinkle with sea salt to serve.

3 RAW SALAD
All but the youngest kale has a harsh texture, and can be unappealing when eaten raw. To soften it, shred it and toss with olive oil and salt, and massage gently for a few minutes before adding to a salad.

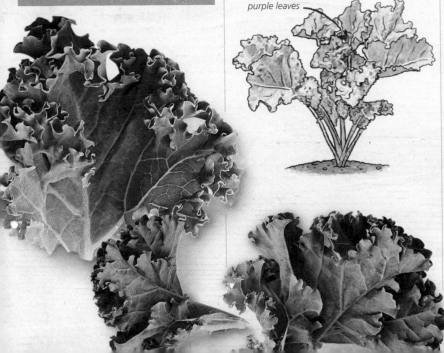

CABBAGE

An excellent source of vitamins K and C, cabbage helps keep your bones, blood, and immune system healthy. Cabbage also contains a host of phytochemicals, which help combat cancer and protect your eyes.

WHY EAT IT?

CANCER PREVENTION
Many studies have shown that people who eat a diet rich in cruciferous vegetables, including cabbage, have a lower risk of developing colon, prostate, and lung cancers.

▼ Savoy cabbage

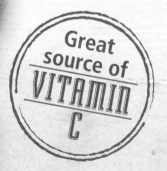

Green-leaved varieties of cabbage are packed with vitamin C

Great source of VITAMIN C

IMMUNE BOOST
The high quantity of vitamin C in cabbage helps to protect the cells that make up the immune system. Vitamin C also boosts the action of white blood cells, helping kill bacteria and viruses.

EYE HEALTH
Cabbage is rich in lutein and zeaxanthin—phytochemicals that can help to reduce the risk of age-related macular degeneration (AMD). High vitamin C content helps protect your eyes from damage by free radicals, potentially reducing the risk of cataracts.

WHAT'S IN IT?

1 cup of raw green cabbage provides an excellent source of vitamins K and C, as well as folate and potassium.

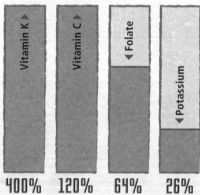

Vitamin K	Vitamin C	Folate	Potassium
400%	120%	64%	26%

Percentage of your daily reference intake

The **vitamin C** in cabbage may help **protect your eyes** from damage by **free radicals, reducing** the risk of **cataracts**.

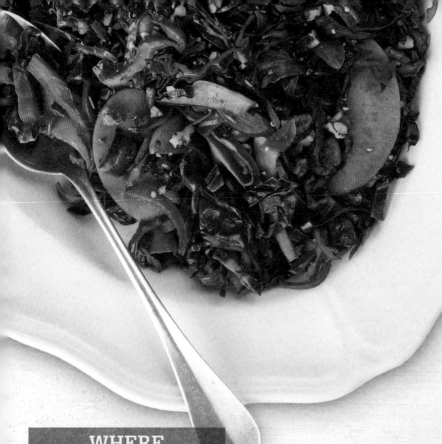

TIP
Brussels sprouts and kohlrabi include some of the same phytochemicals as cabbage, helping combat cancer and protect your eyes.

MAXIMIZE THE BENEFITS

CHOOSE RED AND GREEN
Cabbages with green leaves contain more vitamin K than other varieties, supporting bone strength and healthy blood. Red cabbage contains phytochemicals called anthocyanins, which may help protect against cancer.

EAT IT RAW OR LIGHTLY COOKED
Eat cabbage raw, or cook it only for as long as is necessary, because overcooking leads to a loss of nutrients.

FERMENT IT
Fermented cabbage, such as sauerkraut (see left) and kimchi, is an excellent source of insoluble fiber, which is vital for a healthy digestive tract.

▲ Red cabbage and apple salad

WHERE IS IT FROM?

Cabbages flourish in cool climates, and have been cultivated in Europe since 1000 BCE. Cabbages come in varied colors, such as green, red, and white.

Cabbages are ready to harvest when the heads are firm to the touch

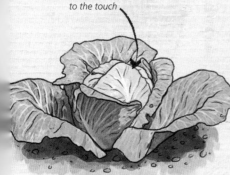

HOW TO EAT IT

1 RED CABBAGE AND APPLE SALAD
Thinly shredded raw cabbage can form a basis for nutritious salads. Try pairing red cabbage with lightly toasted walnuts and thinly sliced apples.

2 SAUERKRAUT
Homemade sauerkraut is simple to make. Massage shredded cabbage with plenty of salt to release natural juices, and leave to ferment at room temperature in a sterilized jar for 3–5 days before serving.

3 ASIAN-STYLE COLESLAW
Red cabbage makes a colorful coleslaw alternative to the classic white variety. Thinly sliced and mixed with red onions, carrot, mint, and cilantro, it can make a deliciously spicy Asian-style 'slaw.

BROCCOLI

An excellent source of bone-strengthening vitamin K and immune-boosting vitamin C, broccoli is also rich in a group of phytochemicals that may help protect against several types of cancer.

WHY EAT IT?

CANCER PREVENTION
Glucosinolates are a group of phytochemicals present in broccoli. Researchers believe that this group helps to protect against cancer in several organs, including the bladder, breasts, colon, liver, lungs, and stomach.

BONE STRENGTH
The high levels of vitamin K in broccoli help bones to absorb calcium. Research suggests that people who consume sufficient quantities of vitamin K may be less likely to develop osteoporosis than those who do not consume enough.

IMMUNE BOOST
Broccoli is an excellent source of vitamin C, which helps to protect the cells that make up the immune system. The vitamin also helps white blood cells to fend off bacteria and viruses.

WHAT'S IN IT?

1 cup of steamed broccoli is an excellent source of vitamins K, C, and B1, as well as folate. Broccoli also contains vitamins A, E, and B2, as well as fiber, niacin, calcium, iron, magnesium, phosphorus, zinc, manganese, and selenium.

Vitamin K	Vitamin C	Folate	Vitamin B1
169%	75%	36%	26%

Percentage of your daily reference intake

Calabrese broccoli ▼

A group of **phytochemicals** present in broccoli may help to **protect** organs against several **types** of **cancer**.

Chlorophyll gives broccoli its color and may help combat cancer

Broccoli stalks are edible and rich in fiber

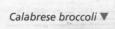

WHERE IS IT FROM?

Broccoli is the head of an edible plant in the cabbage family. It is an annual crop and grows in temperate climates. Native to the land surrounding the Mediterranean, the plant has been popular since the period of the Roman Empire. Calabrese broccoli is the most commonly eaten variety.

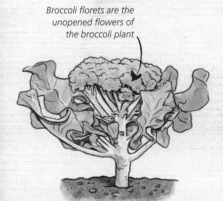

Broccoli florets are the unopened flowers of the broccoli plant

Broccolini ▼

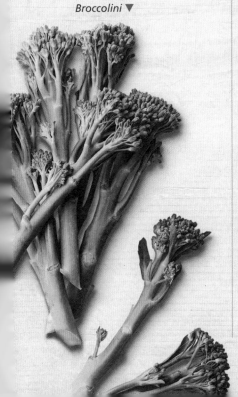

Great source of VITAMIN K

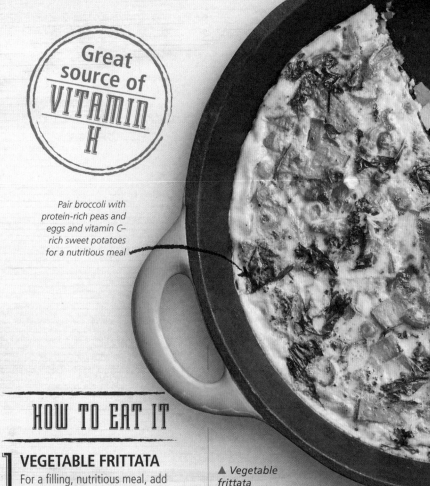

Pair broccoli with protein-rich peas and eggs and vitamin C–rich sweet potatoes for a nutritious meal

▲ *Vegetable frittata*

HOW TO EAT IT

1 VEGETABLE FRITTATA
For a filling, nutritious meal, add broccoli to a simple frittata. Heat a little oil in an ovenproof frying pan and add cooked broccoli, roasted root vegetables, wilted spinach, and beaten egg. Cook for 10–15 minutes and finish under the broiler.

2 SIMPLE SOUP
Finely chopped broccoli takes little time to cook—make a simple soup in less than 10 minutes. Mix with sautéed onions and garlic, add chicken or vegetable stock, and cook for 2–3 minutes before puréeing.

3 ROASTED
Roasting is a great way to bring out the flavor of broccoli. Toss it in a little olive oil, season well, and roast in a hot oven for 20 minutes, until just soft and charred slightly at the edges.

MAXIMIZE THE BENEFITS

TRY DIFFERENT VARIETIES
Broccolini is a variety of broccoli that was developed by crossing broccoli with Chinese kale. It contains higher levels of vitamin C and up to 45 percent more glucosinolates than other types of broccoli. Romanesco broccoli, sometimes know as Roman cauliflower, is not only beautiful but also highly nutritious—it provides impressive amounts of vitamin C, beta-carotene, and vitamin K.

CAULIFLOWER

Cauliflower provides a high quantity of nutrients per calorie—it's rich in fiber, cancer-fighting phytochemicals, and bone-strengthening vitamin K.

WHY EAT IT?

CANCER PREVENTION
Sulforaphane, a phytochemical found in cauliflower, helps prevent cell mutations and blocks enzymes that encourage the spread of cancer cells.

BONE STRENGTH
Cauliflower is a good source of vitamin K, which keeps your bones strong by helping them to absorb calcium. Low intakes of vitamin K have been shown to increase the risk of osteoporosis and bone fractures.

DIGESTIVE HEALTH
With a high water content and plenty of fiber, cauliflower helps to speed the waste materials through your digestive system and prevent constipation.

Unblemished, pale-colored heads are fresh and rich in nutrients

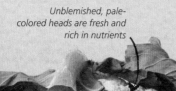

WHAT'S IN IT?

A ¾-cup serving of cauliflower provides a good source of vitamins K and C, as well as folate and potassium.

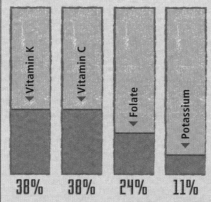

Vitamin K	Vitamin C	Folate	Potassium
38%	38%	24%	11%

Percentage of your daily reference intake

WHERE IS IT FROM?

Part of the cabbage family, cauliflower is a cool-weather crop grown for its globe-shaped flowering head.

Broad leaves protect the heads from damage

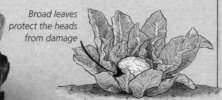

HOW TO EAT IT

1 CAULIFLOWER RICE
Cauliflower makes a nutritious, carbohydrate-free substitute for rice. Simply cut it into florets, discard the core, and process into fine pieces. Stir-fry until al dente or steam in cheesecloth until soft.

2 DAIRY-FREE SAUCE
To make a creamy, dairy-free sauce, cook cauliflower in stock until soft, then purée it with a little olive oil and seasoning until completely smooth.

3 ROAST IT
For a flavorful side dish, toss cauliflower florets in olive oil, season well, and roast in a hot oven until golden brown at the edges but still al dente within.

MAXIMIZE THE BENEFITS

PRESERVE VITAMINS
To reduce the loss of water-soluble vitamins, eat cauliflower raw, steam it in a small amount of water, or use the cooking water in soups or sauces.

SHIITAKE MUSHROOMS

Containing unique phytochemicals, shiitake mushrooms
help control blood pressure and combat cancer.
They are also rich in bone-strengthening copper.

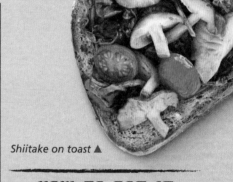

WHY EAT IT?

✓ DISEASE PREVENTION

Shiitake mushrooms contain lentinan, a phytochemical that may help reduce the risk of cancer by preventing healthy cells from developing into cancerous cells. The mushrooms are also believed to have antiviral and antibacterial properties.

BLOOD HEALTH

D-Eritadenine (DEA), a phytochemical found only in shiitake mushrooms, has been found to help your body excrete cholesterol, lowering cholesterol levels.

WHAT'S IN IT?

1 cup of fresh shiitake mushrooms provides an excellent source of copper, as well as selenium and vitamins B2 and B6.

Copper ▲	▲ Selenium	▲ Vitamin B2	▲ Vitamin B6
90%	**45%**	**14%**	**14%**

Percentage of your daily reference intake

Shiitake on toast ▲

HOW TO EAT IT

1 SHIITAKE ON TOAST

Sauté fresh shiitake mushrooms in olive oil with halved cherry tomatoes, baby spinach, and a little garlic. Pile onto freshly toasted whole-wheat bread for a satisfying breakfast or lunch.

2 ADD TO CURRIES

Their strong flavor and meaty texture make shiitake mushrooms a perfect ingredient for a vegetarian curry—try them in coconut milk sauce or in a Thai red curry.

3 FRAGRANT BROTH

Shiitake mushrooms have a deep, earthy flavor that makes an ideal base for a soup, stock, or ramen. Simmer gently with onions and herbs until the broth is dark and fragrant.

WHERE IS IT FROM?

Native to East Asia, shiitake mushrooms grow on the damp, decaying trunks and boughs of deciduous trees.

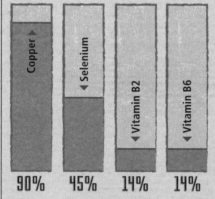

Shiitake mushroom heads can grow up to 8in (20cm) wide

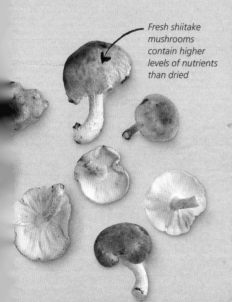

Fresh shiitake mushrooms contain higher levels of nutrients than dried

EGG-FRIED CAULIFLOWER RICE

Packed with cancer-protective phytochemicals and bone-strengthening vitamin K, cauliflower makes a flavorful, carb-free rice substitute in this superfood stir-fry. A rainbow of vegetables supports healthy skin and eyes.

Serves 2 **Prep time** 10 minutes **Cook time** 15 minutes

INGREDIENTS

4 cups **cauliflower** florets, coarsely chopped

a little sunflower oil, for cooking

2 large **eggs**, beaten

1 tbsp coconut oil

1 tsp **sesame oil**

½ cup **carrots**, peeled and finely diced

½ cup red **bell peppers**, finely diced

2 cloves **garlic**, crushed

1 piece of **ginger**, about 2in (5cm), grated

½ cup **edamame** beans

2 tbsp reduced-sodium soy sauce

2 **scallions**, trimmed and finely chopped

2 tbsp **sunflower seeds**

SPECIAL EQUIPMENT

food processor

METHOD

1 Place the cauliflower florets in a food processor and process them until they resemble fine rice. Set aside.

2 Heat a little sunflower oil in a large nonstick frying pan. Pour the beaten egg into the pan and swirl it to make a very large, thin pancake. Cook it over medium heat for 2–3 minutes, just until it sets, then turn it onto a plate and let cool. When the pancake has cooled, roll it up and slice it thinly, then set aside.

3 Heat the coconut and sesame oils in the pan and cook the carrot and bell pepper over medium-high heat for 3–4 minutes until they start to color. Add the garlic, ginger, and edamame and cook for another minute until they are softened, but not brown.

4 Add the cauliflower rice to the pan and stir-fry for another 4–5 minutes, until it has cooked but still has a little crunch to it. Finally, add the soy sauce, chopped egg, scallions, and sunflower seeds, and stir to combine. Serve immediately.

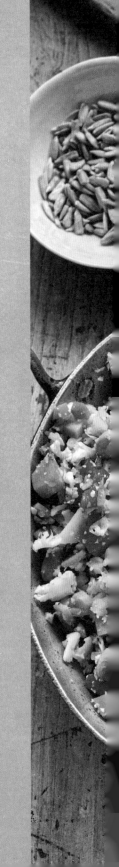

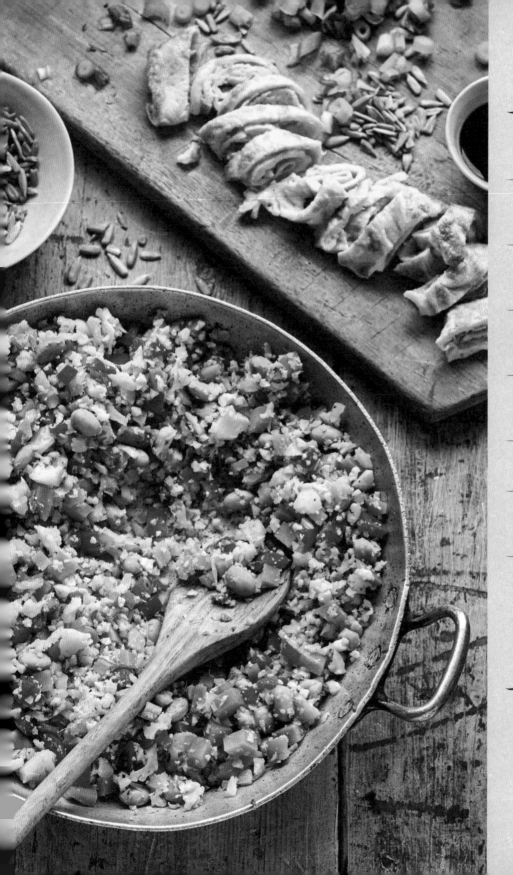

FEATURED SUPERFOODS

CAULIFLOWER
contains **cancer-fighting phytochemicals**

EGGS
help maintain a strong **immune system**

SESAME OIL
may help maintain a **healthy heart**

CARROTS
reduce the risk of certain **types of cancer**

BELL PEPPERS
help maintain **healthy skin**

EDAMAME
may support **eye health**

ONIONS
encourage the growth of **gut-friendly bacteria**

SUNFLOWER SEEDS
help increase **good cholesterol**

Nutrition per serving

Energy 472cals (1877kj)
Carbohydrate 19g
– of which sugars 10.5g
Fiber 8g
Fat 33g
– of which saturated 9g
Salt 1.6g
Protein 20g
Cholesterol 213g

ASPARAGUS

An excellent source of folate, vitamin K, and soluble fiber, asparagus supports circulatory, skeletal, and digestive health, as well as providing important nutrients for women in the early stages of pregnancy.

WHY EAT IT?

DIGESTIVE HEALTH
Asparagus contains a type of fiber called fructooligosaccharides (FOS), which aids digestion by selectively encouraging the growth of friendly bacteria in your gut.

BLOOD HEALTH
Vitamin K and folate, which are both found in generous amounts in asparagus, are needed for the manufacture of red blood cells and for blood clotting. Folate is also an important nutrient for women in the first 12 weeks of pregnancy because it helps protect babies from neural tube defects such as spina bifida.

BONE STRENGTH
The vitamin K present in asparagus also helps bones absorb calcium; studies show that women with high levels of vitamin K in their blood may be less likely to develop osteoporosis.

WHAT'S IN IT?

3½oz (100g, or about 5 fat spears) of lightly steamed asparagus provides a good source of folate and vitamins K, C, and B1. Asparagus also contains vitamins C, A, E, B2, and B6, as well as niacin, fiber, iron, calcium, magnesium, phosphorus, potassium, zinc, copper, and manganese.

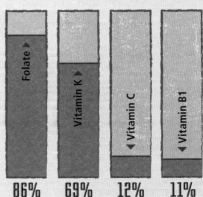

Folate ▲	Vitamin K ▲	◀ Vitamin C	◀ Vitamin B1
86%	**69%**	**12%**	**11%**

Percentage of your daily reference intake

The **high levels** of **vitamin K** and **folate** in asparagus help to keep **red blood cells** healthy.

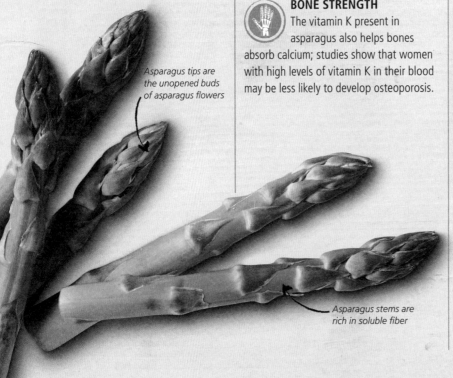

Asparagus tips are the unopened buds of asparagus flowers

Asparagus stems are rich in soluble fiber

WHERE IS IT FROM?

Harvested only after 2 years in the soil, the tender young shoots of asparagus are a prized vegetable. Asparagus grows in wet, temperate climates, and has a short harvesting season. Most varieties are green in color—white asparagus is simply green asparagus that has been grown away from light.

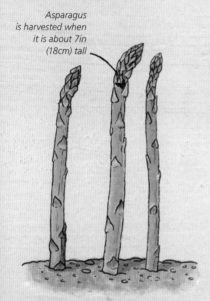

Asparagus is harvested when it is about 7in (18cm) tall

MAXIMIZE THE BENEFITS

GO GREEN

In some parts of the world, white asparagus is considered more of a delicacy than green. Although both varieties are a good source of folate and vitamin K, green asparagus contains higher levels of antioxidant phytochemicals, including rutin and chlorophyll.

HOW TO EAT IT

1 STEAM IT

Lightly steam asparagus to preserve its nutrients and delicate texture. For a light dinner, toss steamed asparagus with cooked chicken, radicchio, and grilled red bell peppers, and dress with a little lemon juice and olive oil.

2 IN A FRITTATA

Finely sliced asparagus makes a beautiful frittata. Sauté it with garlic and handfuls of fresh herbs, then bind together with whisked eggs and bake until just set.

Grilled asparagus salad ▶

3 GRILLED ASPARAGUS SALAD

For a nutrient-rich side dish, toss asparagus spears in olive oil and grill for about 10 minutes, until al dente. Mix with chopped tomato, basil, and dill.

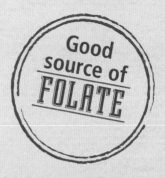

Good source of FOLATE

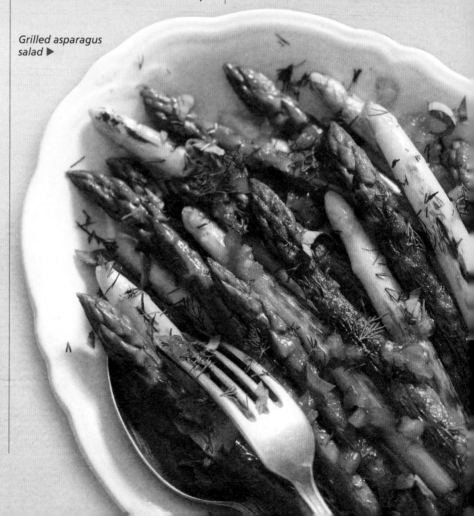

BEANS

Beans are rich in cancer-fighting vitamin C, energy-boosting B vitamins, and gut-healthy fiber, as well as phytochemicals that help keep your eyes healthy. Fava and green beans are rich in fiber, and edamame beans are packed with protein.

WHY EAT IT?

DIGESTIVE HEALTH
All fresh beans are a good source of fiber, but fava beans contain around twice as much fiber as other beans. Insoluble fiber, the type in fava beans, speeds the passage of waste material through the gut and helps reduce the risk of constipation, hemorrhoids, diverticular disease, and colorectal and breast cancers.

BONE STRENGTH
Beans are rich in vitamin K, which helps the bones use calcium. People who have a low intake of vitamin K have been shown to have a greater risk of bone fractures and osteoporosis. Vitamin K also helps your blood to clot properly.

EYE HEALTH
The phytochemicals lutein and zeaxanthin, as well as carotenoid compounds, found in beans help to protect your eyes from damage by free radicals, which can increase the risk of age-related macular degeneration (AMD) and cataracts.

WHAT'S IN IT?

½ cup of cooked fava beans are a good source of vitamin C, fiber, niacin, and folate. Fava beans contain more fiber than other varieties of bean. They also contain vitamins A, B2, and K, as well as iron.

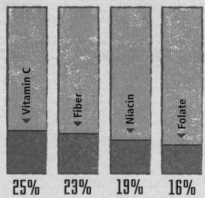

Vitamin C	Fiber	Niacin	Folate
25%	23%	19%	16%

Percentage of your daily reference intake

Vitamin K–rich beans help to strengthen bones against **fractures** and **osteoporosis**.

Green beans ▶

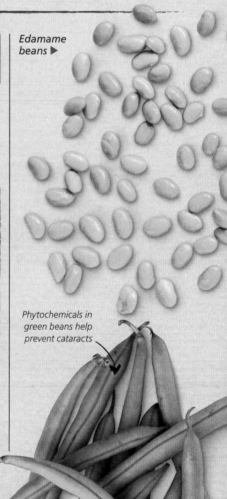

Edamame beans ▶

Phytochemicals in green beans help prevent cataracts

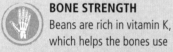

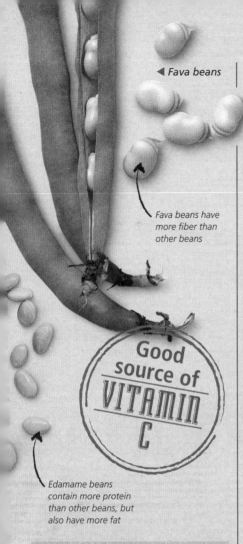

◀ Fava beans

Fava beans have more fiber than other beans

Good source of VITAMIN C

Edamame beans contain more protein than other beans, but also have more fat

HOW TO EAT IT

1 SUPERFOOD PASTA
Give traditional pasta primavera a superfood twist. Blanch handfuls of fava beans and sliced green beans, then combine them with spiralized zucchini and fresh pesto.

2 EDAMAME DIP
Frozen, shelled edamame beans can be whipped up into a simple, nourishing dip in minutes. Purée blanched and cooled beans with a little Greek yogurt and mint for a lighter alternative to hummus.

3 GREEN BEAN STIR-FRY
Cook green beans in a tasty, nutrient-laden stir-fry along with nutty buckwheat noodles, bean sprouts, broccoli, fennel, dried shredded coconut, sesame seeds, cashews, and plenty of ginger and garlic.

Beans are a great source of the **insoluble fiber** that keeps your **digestive system healthy** and helps it remove **cancer-causing toxins**.

Lightly frying in oil helps your body absorb the beans' nutrients

MAXIMIZE THE BENEFITS

COOK WITH STEAM
To preserve the levels of C and B vitamins in beans, cook them lightly. Steam the beans in a small amount of water until they are just tender.

COOK OR SERVE WITH OIL
Serving beans with a small amount of oil will make it easier for the body to absorb the phytochemicals that help to protect your eyes from damage by free radicals.

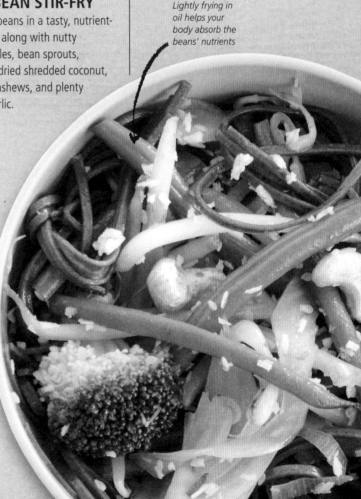

Green bean stir-fry ▶

DRIED LEGUMES

Dried legumes, including beans and peas, support your digestive and heart health with soluble and insoluble fiber. They also provide protein, energy-boosting manganese and folate, and disease-fighting phytochemicals.

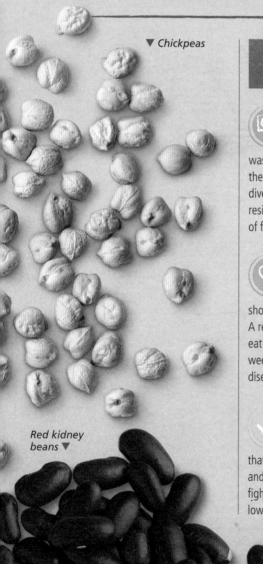

▼ *Chickpeas*

Red kidney beans ▼

WHY EAT IT?

DIGESTIVE HEALTH
Legumes are rich in insoluble fiber, the type that helps move waste through the gut, and thereby lowers the risk of constipation, hemorrhoids, and diverticular disease. They are also high in resistant starch, which supports the growth of friendly bacteria in the lower gut.

HEART HEALTH
Dried legumes are a good source of soluble fiber, which has been shown to help reduce bad LDL cholesterol. A recent U.S. study found that people who eat beans and pulses four or more times a week have a 22 percent lower risk of heart disease than those who don't.

DISEASE PREVENTION
Beans contain isoflavones, estrogen-like phytochemicals that are linked to a reduced risk of breast and prostate cancers, and cholesterol-fighting phytosterols, which may help lower the risk of heart disease.

Red kidney beans are rich in manganese, which helps your body produce energy

WHAT'S IN IT?

½ cup of cooked red kidney beans provides a good source of manganese, folate, potassium, and iron. Red kidney beans also contain vitamins B1 and B2, as well as protein and fiber. They contain similar nutrients to other dried legumes.

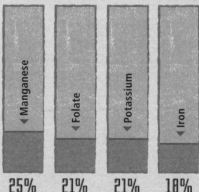

| Manganese | Folate | Potassium | Iron |
| 25% | 21% | 21% | 18% |

Percentage of your daily reference intake

▼ *Navy beans*

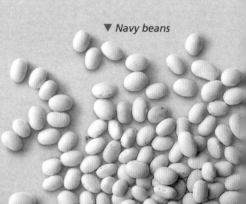

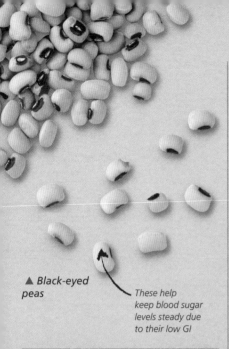

▲ Black-eyed peas

These help keep blood sugar levels steady due to their low GI

HOW TO EAT IT

1 IN SALAD
Bean salad has a slightly old-fashioned reputation, but it can be delicious and nutritious. Cook your own mixed beans, then dress with plenty of olive oil, lemon juice, and handfuls of fresh herbs.

2 BEAN SOUP
Cook plenty of onions and garlic in olive oil, then add canned tomatoes and soaked, dried beans or canned beans and flavor with a little chopped rosemary. Cook until the beans are softened.

3 CHICKPEA FRITTERS
Make flavorful fritters using drained and coarsely mashed canned chickpeas and chopped mixed vegetables. Bind with an egg, season well, and pan-fry. Serve with a yogurt and herb dip.

Eating **dried legumes four or more** times a week may **lower** the **risk** of **heart disease** by nearly a **quarter**.

Chickpea fritters ▼

Black beans ▲

Good source of **MANGANESE**

Chickpeas make a protein-rich base for simple fritters

MAXIMIZE THE BENEFITS

CHOOSE DRIED OR CANNED
Both dried and canned legumes offer similar levels of nutrients. Most dried legumes need soaking before cooking and have a long cooking time. Canned beans may be time-saving, but choose those without added sugar or salt, and rinse well to remove sugars that can cause flatulence.

COOK WITH HERBS AND SPICES
If you're using dried beans, change the water several times during soaking, and cook them with turmeric, cumin, ginger, fennel, or sage to help reduce flatulence. Serve with vitamin-C-rich foods to help the body absorb iron from the beans.

Navy beans are high in protein but very low in fat

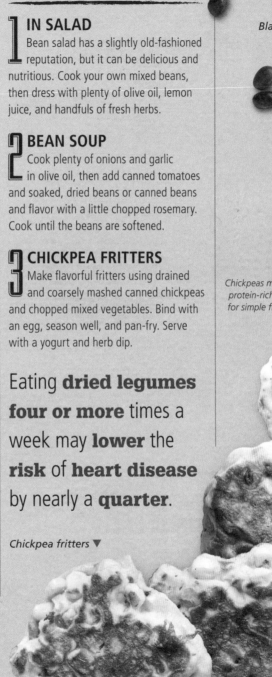

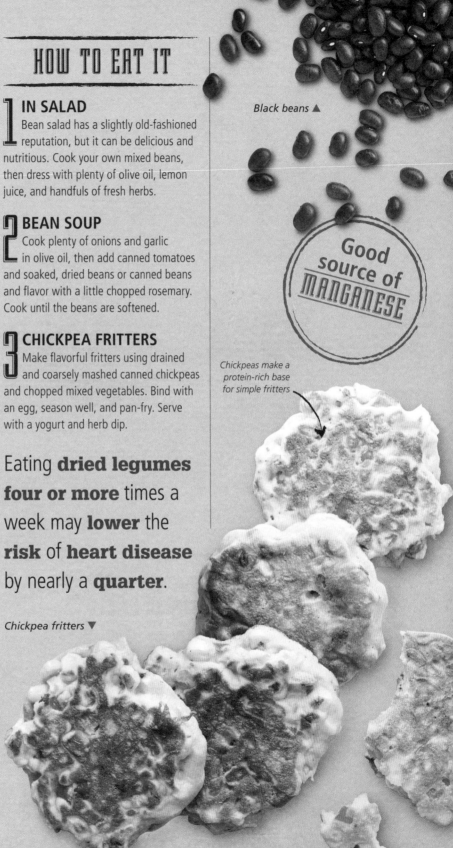

PEAS

Containing fiber, folate, and vitamins A, C, and K, peas support your digestive, nervous, and circulatory systems. They are a particularly useful superfood for those who follow a vegetarian diet, as they are high in protein and iron.

WHY EAT IT?

DIGESTIVE HEALTH
Peas are a good source of soluble and insoluble fiber—both of which are important for a healthy gut. Varieties eaten with their pod, such as sugar snap and snow peas, contain more fiber than podded peas.

BLOOD HEALTH
Peas are a good source of iron, particularly useful for people who don't eat meat. They are also a good source of folate, which is needed for the manufacture of red blood cells.

HEART HEALTH
Peas contain both soluble fiber and a phytochemical called beta-sitosterol—these work together to help reduce bad cholesterol. Research shows that eating 4½oz (125g) of legumes (peas, chickpeas, beans, and lentils) a day could reduce bad cholesterol by up to 5 percent.

The **soluble fiber** and **phytochemicals** in peas work together to help **reduce bad cholesterol**; research shows that **adding more legumes** to your **diet** could reduce bad cholesterol by **up to 5 percent**.

Peas, such as sugar snaps, that are eaten in the pod are an excellent source of fiber

WHAT'S IN IT?

¾ cup of peas, boiled from frozen, are a good source of vitamin B1, folate, fiber, and iron. Peas also contain vitamins A, E, B2, B6, and K, as well as protein, niacin, biotin, potassium, calcium, phosphorus, magnesium, zinc, and copper.

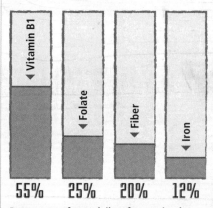

Vitamin B1	Folate	Fiber	Iron
55%	25%	20%	12%

Percentage of your daily reference intake

Fresh, nutrient-rich peas should be plump and evenly colored

WHERE IS IT FROM?

Native to the eastern Mediterranean region, peas are now grown in temperate regions around the world. They are part of the legume family, along with beans and lentils. In botanical terms, peas are considered to be a fruit, as the seeds develop from the ovary of the pea flower. Garden or green peas must be removed from their pods before eating; snow peas and sugar snap peas have been bred to have tender, edible pods.

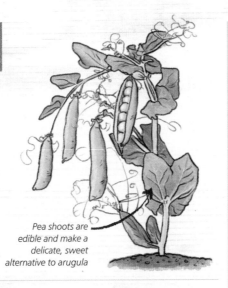

Pea shoots are edible and make a delicate, sweet alternative to arugula

MAXIMIZE THE BENEFITS

EAT THEM QUICKLY
Fresh peas are sweet and flavorful, but can be tricky to get ahold of because they have a short growing season. If you do manage to source some, eat them as soon as possible—the levels of vitamins in the peas start to decline right after harvest.

FROZEN BENEFITS
Frozen peas are just as nutritious as fresh peas. In fact, studies show that they often contain more vitamin C than fresh peas, because they are frozen within hours of being harvested, which helps to preserve vitamins.

HOW TO EAT IT

1 BRAISED GREENS
Highlight fresh peas' natural sweetness by braising them in stock with onions, garlic, and some quartered Little Gem lettuces. Serve as a light side dish.

2 MAKE A PESTO
Minted pea pesto makes a quick and healthy topping for bruschetta. Blend cooked and cooled peas with a handful of mint, half a clove of crushed garlic, and a little olive oil, until almost smooth.

3 MIXED VEGETABLE SPAGHETTINI
Add pockets of sweetness to a simple vegetable pasta with a handful of fresh petite peas. Simply add the peas in with the nearly cooked pasta for the last 2–3 minutes of cooking time.

Mixed vegetable spaghettini ▶

Good source of VITAMIN B1

Podded peas add protein and a hint of sweetness to a simple pasta dish

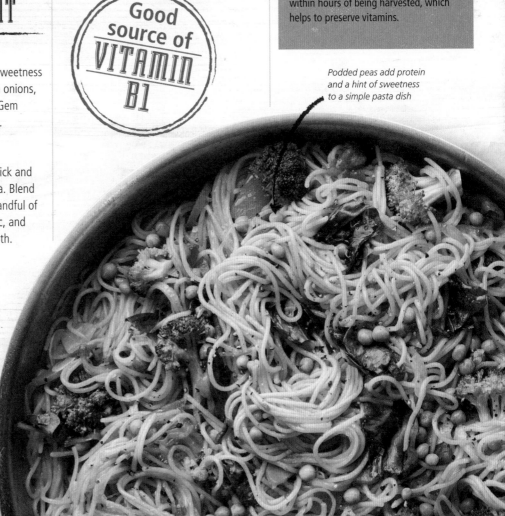

LENTILS

All types of lentils are rich in cholesterol-lowering fiber. They are also a low-fat source of iron, vital for the cardiovascular system and for energy, and contain B vitamins that protect against heart disease.

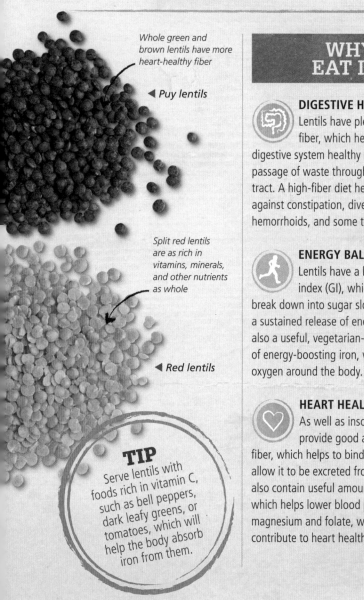

Whole green and brown lentils have more heart-healthy fiber

◀ *Puy lentils*

Split red lentils are as rich in vitamins, minerals, and other nutrients as whole

◀ *Red lentils*

TIP
Serve lentils with foods rich in vitamin C, such as bell peppers, dark leafy greens, or tomatoes, which will help the body absorb iron from them.

WHY EAT IT?

DIGESTIVE HEALTH
Lentils have plenty of insoluble fiber, which helps to keep the digestive system healthy by speeding the passage of waste through the digestive tract. A high-fiber diet helps protect against constipation, diverticular disease, hemorrhoids, and some types of cancer.

ENERGY BALANCE
Lentils have a low glycemic index (GI), which means they break down into sugar slowly, providing a sustained release of energy. Lentils are also a useful, vegetarian-friendly source of energy-boosting iron, which transports oxygen around the body.

HEART HEALTH
As well as insoluble fiber, lentils provide good amounts of soluble fiber, which helps to bind cholesterol and allow it to be excreted from the body. They also contain useful amounts of potassium, which helps lower blood pressure, and magnesium and folate, which also contribute to heart health.

WHAT'S IN IT?

A ½-cup serving of cooked green lentils provides a useful source of selenium, manganese, copper, and iron. All lentils contain these nutrients. They also contain vitamins B1, B2, and B6, as well as magnesium, folate, calcium, and protein.

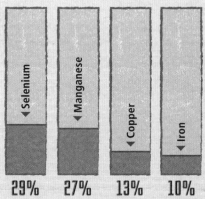

Selenium · Manganese · Copper · Iron

29%   **27%**   **13%**   **10%**

Percentage of your daily reference intake

Fiber in lentils helps protect against **constipation**, **diverticular disease**, and some **cancers**.

All lentils provide **soluble fiber**, which contributes to reducing cholesterol. They also contain **potassium**, which helps **lower high blood pressure**, and **magnesium** and **folate**, which are good for the heart.

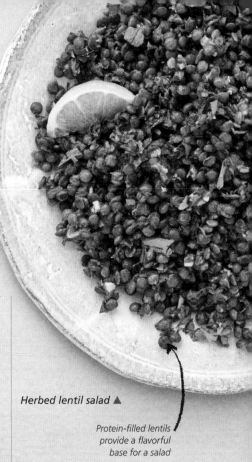

Herbed lentil salad ▲

Protein-filled lentils provide a flavorful base for a salad

WHERE IS IT FROM?

Lentils, thought to have originated in central Asia, are one of the first foods to have been cultivated. Grown around the world in the tropics and temperate zones, they are harvested for the edible seeds. Sometimes eaten fresh but more often dried, lentils belong to the group of legumes known as pulses, which also includes dried peas and beans. Dozens of varieties are cultivated. The most common types are green or brown, but they are also available in yellow, black, red, and orange. They are sold whole or split into halves.

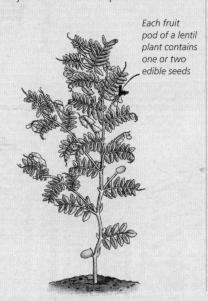

Each fruit pod of a lentil plant contains one or two edible seeds

HOW TO EAT IT

1 HERBED LENTIL SALAD
Some lentils, such as red, collapse on cooking. Cook a firmer variety, such as beluga or Puy, for a salad. Puy lentils, which are green, come from the Le Puy region of France, and have a unique peppery flavor. Beluga lentils, tiny and round, are named for the caviar they resemble. Dress the salad while still warm with a red wine vinaigrette and plenty of chopped herbs.

2 LENTIL PILAF
Adding lentils to cooked rice gives a side dish a burst of extra color, as well as boosting nutritional value. Try mixing whole-grain rice with lentils, and stir-frying with onions, garlic, and ginger. For extra flavor, add a cardamom pod and cinnamon stick to the stir-fry, and remove before serving.

3 DHAL
Dhal is a great standby dish for softer varieties of lentils, such as yellow or red. Cook them slowly in coconut milk with a little ginger and garlic, and flavor with garam masala and turmeric. Don't let the coconut milk boil, or it will curdle. Serve with rice and a little yogurt.

MAXIMIZE THE BENEFITS

USE DRIED
Unlike other pulses, lentils don't need to be soaked before cooking, so buy dried lentils (rather than canned lentils) and cook from scratch for maximum nutrients.

RINSE CANNED
Canned lentils, a good pantry standby, retain most of their nutrients, but salt is sometimes added during processing. The process also adds sugars that can cause flatulence, so rinse canned lentils well before using.

PUY LENTIL & MUSHROOM BURGERS

These vegan burgers are more nutrient-rich than traditional beef burgers. Puy lentils are rich in soluble fiber, which stabilizes your blood sugar and makes you feel full for longer, while onions contribute probiotic fiber.

Serves 4   **Prep time** 15 minutes, plus cooling and chilling   **Cook time** 40–45 minutes

INGREDIENTS

1/2 cup Puy **lentils**

3 tbsp olive oil, plus extra for cooking the burgers

1 **onion**, finely chopped

1lb (450g) portobello mushrooms, wiped, trimmed, and coarsely chopped

2 cloves **garlic**, crushed

1 tsp fresh **thyme** leaves, chopped

1 tbsp finely chopped flat-leaf **parsley**

1 tbsp balsamic vinegar

1/2 cup fresh white breadcrumbs

1 tbsp **nutritional yeast**

salt and freshly ground black pepper

SPECIAL EQUIPMENT

food processor

METHOD

1 Place the lentils in a saucepan of cold water and bring to a boil. Reduce to a low simmer, skimming any foam off the top, and cook for 15 minutes until they are just soft. Drain and rinse the lentils, then set aside to cool.

2 Heat 1 tablespoon of the oil in a large, nonstick frying pan. Cook the onion over medium heat for 5 minutes, until softened but not brown. Add the remaining oil and the chopped mushrooms, and cook for another 15–20 minutes, until they break down and there is no moisture left in the pan. Add the garlic, thyme, and parsley and cook for another minute, until the garlic is fragrant. Add the balsamic vinegar and remove from the heat.

3 Put the mushroom mixture, cooled lentils, breadcrumbs, and nutritional yeast into a food processor and season well. Pulse carefully until it is just mixed and still has some texture.

4 Let the mixture cool for 5 minutes. Shape the cooled mixture into four equal-sized patties and chill, covered, for 30 minutes to allow them to firm up.

5 Clean the frying pan with paper towels. Heat a little oil in the pan and cook the burgers over medium heat for 3–4 minutes on each side, until they are well browned and cooked through. Serve immediately in whole-grain bread buns, with your choice of accompaniments.

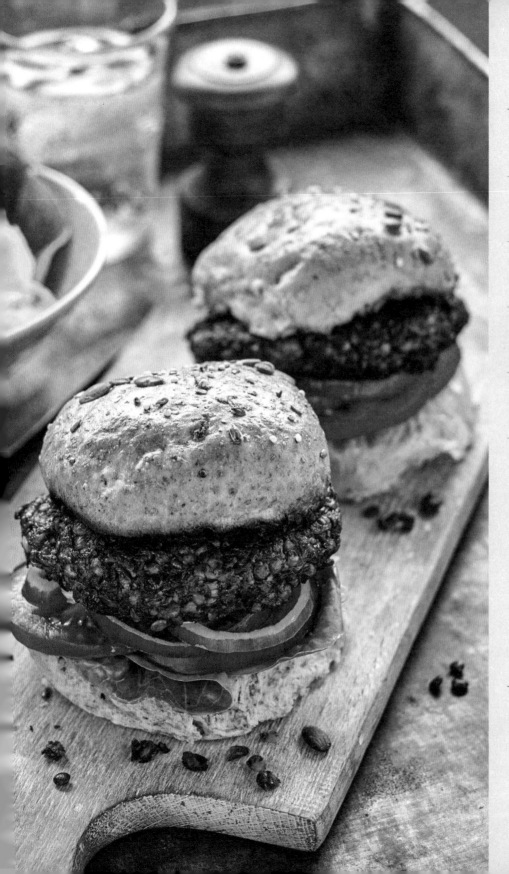

FEATURED SUPERFOODS

LENTILS
help stabilize **blood sugar**
and reduce **cholesterol**

ONIONS
encourage the growth
of **gut-friendly bacteria**

GARLIC
may deactivate
cancer-causing agents

THYME
may help lower
blood pressure

PARSLEY
helps maintain
healthy bones

NUTRITIONAL YEAST
helps to keep your
blood healthy

Nutrition
per serving

Energy 450cals (1793kj)

Carbohydrate 59g
– of which sugars 6.5g

Fiber 10g

Fat 14g
– of which saturated 2g

Salt 1g

Protein 11g

Cholesterol 0g

BELL PEPPERS

Bell peppers are an incredible source of vitamins C and A, which support your skin and immune system. They also provide beneficial carotenoid compounds such as beta-carotene, which has been shown to reduce the risk of certain cancers.

WHY EAT IT?

SKIN HEALTH

Vitamin C is essential for the manufacture of collagen, which is a protein necessary for healthy bones, teeth, gums, capillaries, and connective tissue. A powerful antioxidant, vitamin C also helps to neutralize free radicals that can accelerate skin aging. Bell peppers also contain beta-carotene, which your body converts into vitamin A to help keep skin healthy.

IMMUNE BOOST

Vitamin C helps to protect the cells that make up the immune system, and boosts the action of bacteria- and virus-combating white blood cells.

CANCER PREVENTION

Diets rich in beta-carotene and other carotenoids are known to reduce the risk of certain types of cancer, including lung cancer. Bell peppers are naturally rich in these compounds, making them a safer source of beta-carotene than supplements, which some studies suggest may increase the risk of certain cancers.

WHAT'S IN IT?

1 cup of raw red bell pepper provides an excellent source of vitamins C and A, as well as copper and vitamin B6. Peppers also contain vitamins E, B1, and B2, as well as fiber, niacin, folate, iron, magnesium, phosphorus, and potassium.

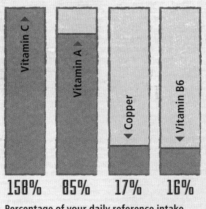

Vitamin C ▸	Vitamin A ▸	◂ Copper	◂ Vitamin B6
158%	85%	17%	16%

Percentage of your daily reference intake

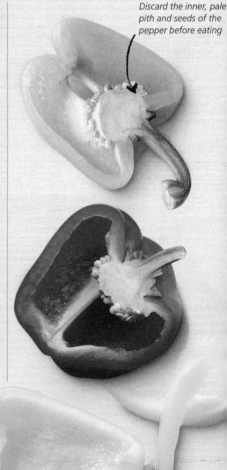

Discard the inner, pale pith and seeds of the pepper before eating

Glossy, firm-skinned bell peppers with bright green stems are fresh and rich in nutrients

WHERE IS IT FROM?

Native to Mexico and Central America, bell peppers are part of a group of flowering plants in the nightshade family, which includes potatoes and eggplant. Columbus brought bell peppers from the Americas to Europe in the fifteenth century. All peppers, including chiles, belong to the *capsicum* genus.

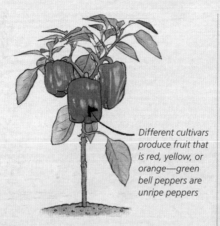

Different cultivars produce fruit that is red, yellow, or orange—green bell peppers are unripe peppers

MAXIMIZE THE BENEFITS

CHOOSE RED
Bell peppers come in a variety of colors, but red bell peppers pack the biggest punch in terms of nutrition—they contain 11 times more beta-carotene and 1½ times more vitamin C than green bell peppers.

EAT RAW OR WITH OIL
To get the most vitamin C, eat bell peppers raw. Cooking or serving them with some oil helps the body absorb the carotenoids.

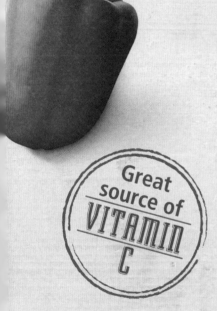

HOW TO EAT IT

1 STUFFED PEPPERS
Fill seeded bell pepper halves with cooked rice or buckwheat, crack an egg into each, and bake in a medium oven for 8–10 minutes, until the egg is just set.

2 MUHAMMARA
Eat this Middle Eastern dip with crudités or broiled fish. Blend roasted, skinned red bell peppers with toasted walnuts, pomegranate molasses, and seasoning.

3 PEPERONATA
A classic Italian dish, peperonata is a true taste of summer. Cook strips of red and yellow bell peppers with onion, garlic, and chopped ripe tomatoes, until soft and unctuous. Season and serve with diced boiled potatoes and black olives.

Peperonata ▶

Great source of VITAMIN C

Red bell peppers contain **11 times** more **beta-carotene** and **1.5 times** more **vitamin C** than green bell peppers.

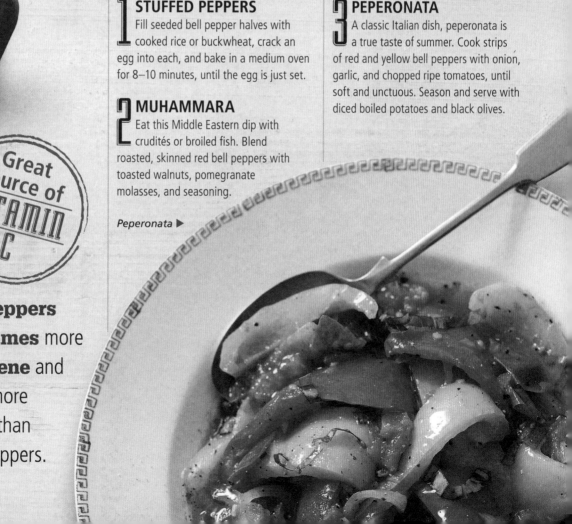

TOMATOES

Rich in a group of phytochemicals called carotenoids, tomatoes may help reduce the risk of heart disease and stroke, and provide protection against cancer. Tomatoes are also a good source of immune-boosting vitamin C.

WHY EAT IT?

HEART HEALTH

Lycopene, a bright red carotenoid found in tomatoes, may help protect your heart. Research suggests that men with high levels of lycopene in their blood are up to 50 percent less likely to have a heart attack compared with men who have low levels of lycopene. Tomatoes also contain a group of phytochemicals called flavonoids, which have been linked to a reduced risk of heart disease.

CANCER PREVENTION

The carotenoid lycopene in tomatoes may help prevent cancer. Studies suggest that diets rich in lycopene offer protection against cancers of the prostate, stomach, and colon. Experts believe that lycopene may inhibit—and possibly even reverse—the growth of cancerous tumors.

SKIN HEALTH

Tomatoes are rich in beta-carotene, a carotenoid that is converted into vitamin A after it has been digested. Vitamin A is a vital nutrient that helps maintain skin health, and protects your eyes against damage by free radicals. Beta-carotene also helps to improve the tone and color of your skin.

The **carotenoids** in tomatoes may help **reduce** the risk of **heart disease** by up to **50 percent**.

WHAT'S IN IT?

1 medium tomato (2½oz/75g) provides a good source of vitamin C, folate, potassium, and vitamin K. Tomatoes also contain manganese.

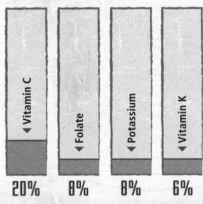

▼Vitamin C	▼Folate	▼Potassium	▼Vitamin K
20%	8%	8%	6%

Percentage of your daily reference intake

Good source of VITAMIN C

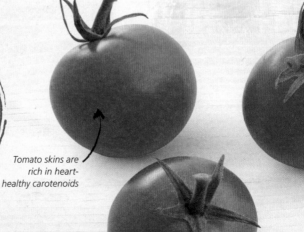

Tomato skins are rich in heart-healthy carotenoids

WHERE IS IT FROM?

Originating in highland coastal regions of South America, tomatoes were cultivated by the Aztecs and Mayans. Tomatoes are the fruit of a flowering plant in the nightshade family. There are over 5,000 varieties of tomato, which are cultivated in temperate climates across the world.

The fruits of different varieties are red, orange, yellow, and purple

MAXIMIZE THE BENEFITS

EAT RAW, COOKED, OR CANNED
Fresh tomatoes have higher levels of vitamin C and folate than cooked or canned tomatoes. However, cooking tomatoes makes it easier for your body to absorb heart-healthy lycopene.

PAIR WITH AVOCADO OR BROCCOLI
Your body absorbs up to 44 times more heart-healthy lycopene from tomatoes if you eat them with avocados. Studies also show that eating tomatoes with broccoli maximizes their cancer-fighting effects.

TRY DIFFERENT VARIETIES
Cherry tomatoes contain high levels of antioxidant flavonoids, purple varieties are rich in anthocyanins, and yellow tomatoes contain high levels of blood-healthy folate.

HOW TO EAT IT

1 SIMPLE SALAD
Make the most of the summer's bounty with a bright salad containing as many different varieties of tomatoes as you can find, sliced and dressed simply with olive oil and torn basil leaves.

2 IN PASTA
For a simple lunch or dinner, pan-fry halved cherry tomatoes in olive oil with a little garlic, then toss with cooked whole-wheat fusilli and blanched broccoli florets. Season with salt and pepper and eat immediately.

3 TOMATO CONSOMMÉ
Tomato consommé has all the flavor and benefits of ripe tomatoes in a delicate, clear broth. Blend fresh tomatoes with aromatics such as fresh dill, basil, tarragon, or chives, and let strain through cheesecloth overnight. Season to taste with salt, pepper, sherry vinegar, and a little olive oil, and serve chilled.

Tomato consommé ▶

Tomatoes are rich in **lycopene**, a **phytochemical** that supports **heart health**. Your body absorbs up to **44 times more** lycopene from tomatoes when you **eat them with avocado**.

Using tomatoes raw maximizes the levels of immune-boosting vitamin C

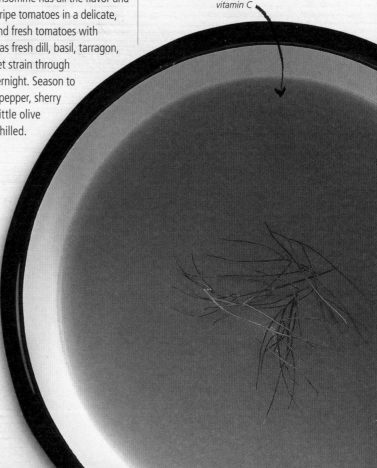

AVOCADOS

The avocado is technically a fruit, but is usually used as a vegetable. It contains almost 20 different vitamins and minerals, phytochemicals, and good fats that together support your heart health and nervous system.

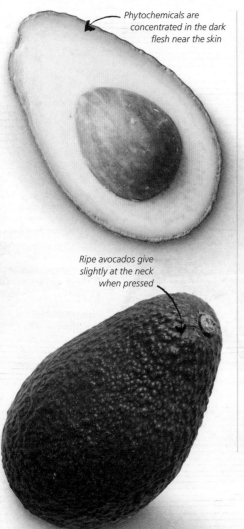

Phytochemicals are concentrated in the dark flesh near the skin

Ripe avocados give slightly at the neck when pressed

WHY EAT IT?

HEART HEALTH
Avocados contain a trio of heart-healthy nutrients. Vitamin E helps prevent the oxidation of LDL cholesterol, potassium can help reduce high blood pressure by counteracting the effect of salt, and beta-sitosterol (a phytochemical) helps maintain healthy cholesterol levels.

EYE HEALTH
Lutein, a phytochemical found in avocados, helps protect your eyes from damage by free radicals and reduces the risk of cataracts and age-related macular degeneration (AMD).

BRAIN POWER
Avocados provide vitamin B6, which is important for a healthy nervous system. Low levels of vitamin B6 in the blood have been linked with depression and chronic fatigue syndrome.

WHAT'S IN IT?

1 small avocado (3½oz/100g) provides good quantities of vitamins E and B6, as well as potassium and copper. It also contains vitamins C, B1, B2, and K, as well as niacin, manganese, iron, zinc, magnesium, and phosphorus.

Vitamin E	Vitamin B6	Potassium	Copper
27%	26%	22%	19%

Percentage of your daily reference intake

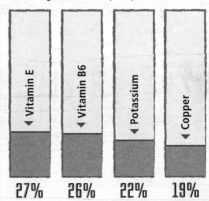

The buttery flesh contains healthy monosaturated fats

WHERE IS IT FROM?

Avocado is the fruit of a flowering tree in the *Lauraceae* family. Native to Central America and the Caribbean, it has long been an important part of the Mexican diet. There are more than 1,000 cultivars of avocado, with shapes ranging from round to pear-shaped, and skin colors ranging from green to purple.

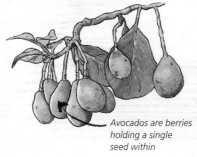

Avocados are berries holding a single seed within

HOW TO PREPARE

Using a large knife, cut around the avocado vertically, working the knife around the pit. Twist the two halves apart to separate them. Strike the cutting edge of the knife into the pit, then twist and lift the knife to remove the pit from the flesh.

Twist the knife as you lift it to release the pit

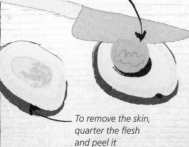

To remove the skin, quarter the flesh and peel it

HOW TO EAT IT

1 SALSA
Make a zingy, heart-healthy salsa with diced avocado, diced tomato, and fresh corn. Serve with any grilled fish and a mixed leaf salad for an eye-catching dish.

2 GREEN SMOOTHIE
Avocados work especially well in green smoothies with kale or spinach. Its creamy texture makes a great dairy substitute—just add half an avocado, coarsely chopped, in place of yogurt or kefir for a dairy-free breakfast smoothie.

3 AVOCADO TOASTS
For a snack or light lunch, pile up sliced avocado with other superfoods, such as cashew butter, cherry tomatoes, slivers of nori, and a sprinkling of sesame seeds.

TIP
If you have unripe avocados, speed up the ripening process by placing them in a brown paper bag with an apple or a banana.

Toss avocado in lime or lemon juice to prevent it from oxidizing and getting brown

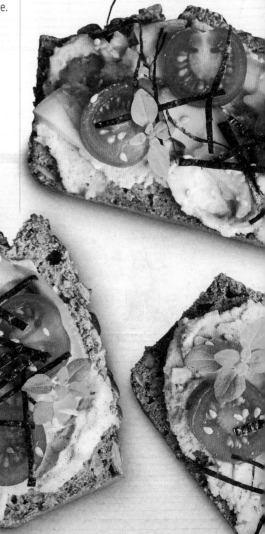

Avocado toasts ▶

CACAO & AVOCADO MOUSSE

This simple dessert provides all the rich taste of the most decadent chocolate mousse, without the cream, butter, or processed sugar. Avocados are full of antioxidant phytochemicals, and cacao may help lower blood pressure.

Serves 4 **Prep time** 5 minutes, plus chilling

INGREDIENTS

5 ripe **avocados**, coarsely chopped, about 3 cups in total

6 tbsp raw **cacao** powder

¼ cup honey or maple syrup

1 tsp vanilla extract

¼ cup **almond** or coconut milk

cacao nibs, to serve

SPECIAL EQUIPMENT

food processor

METHOD

1 To make the mousse, place all the ingredients, except the cacao nibs, into a food processor and process them until completely smooth, adding a little extra almond or coconut milk if necessary.

2 Pour the mixture into a serving dish or four 5fl oz (150ml) glasses. Refrigerate for at least 1 hour, until chilled. To serve, sprinkle the mousse with cacao nibs.

SUPER SWAP

- Add natural peanut butter for energy-boosting B vitamins
- Top with sleep-regulating chopped dried cherries or heart-healthy pistachios

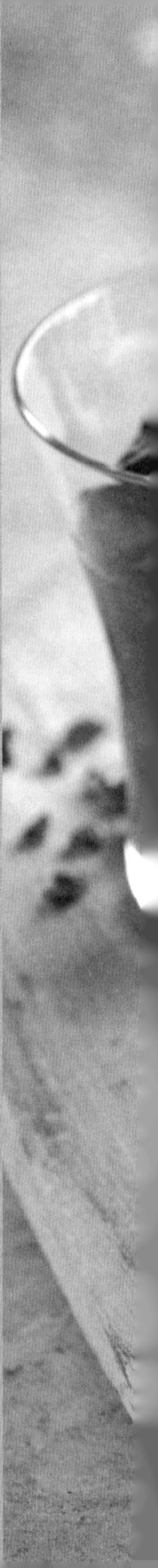

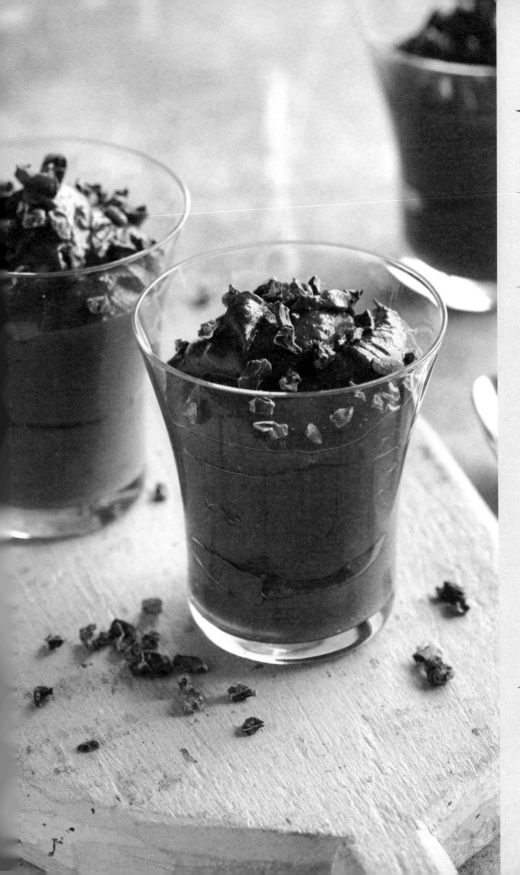

FEATURED
SUPERFOODS

AVOCADOS
help maintain healthy
cholesterol levels and
protect your **heart**

CACAO
may help lower
blood pressure
and protect against
heart disease

ALMONDS
reduce the risk of
heart disease

Nutrition
per serving

Energy 290cals (1142kj)
Carbohydrate 18g
– of which sugars 16g
Fiber 6g
Fat 21g
– of which saturated 5g
Salt 0g
Protein 4g
Cholesterol 0g

BROWN SEAWEED

Brown seaweeds, such as wakame and kombu, are a rare, exceptionally rich source of the mineral iodine, which helps regulate your hormones. Brown seaweeds are also a good source of gut-healthy fiber.

WHY EAT IT?

HIGH IN IODINE

All brown seaweeds contain very high levels of iodine, with wakame and kombu containing the highest quantities. Iodine is an important mineral that helps maintain your thyroid gland, which produces and regulates hormones. Even a marginal iodine deficiency can cause a number of health problems including fatigue, muscle weakness, depression, weight problems, and increased cholesterol levels. It is possible, but rare, to consume too much iodine—do not consume more than 800mg per day on a regular basis.

DIGESTIVE HEALTH

Alginate, which is found in brown seaweed, has been shown to protect the gut and slow down digestion. Research also shows that people who regularly eat seaweed regularly have higher levels of good bacteria in their gut.

BLOOD HEALTH

Brown seaweeds are a rich source of folate, which helps your body manufacture red blood cells. Early research has shown that wakame may help prevent high blood pressure and stroke.

WHAT'S IN IT?

3½oz (100g) of wakame is an excellent source of iodine, folate, manganese, and magnesium. Wakame contains more iodine than any other variety of brown seaweed.

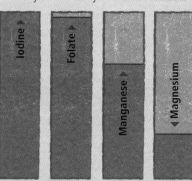

Iodine	Folate	Manganese	Magnesium
8666%	98%	70%	28%

Percentage of your daily reference intake

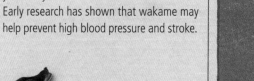

Wakame is usually sold dried, in small pieces

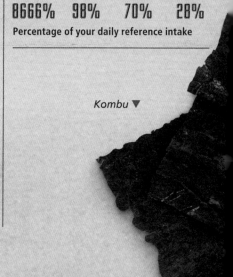

Kombu ▼

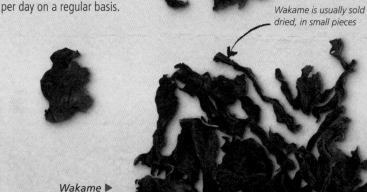

Wakame ▶

Iodine-rich kombu adds flavor to a broth for ramen

WHERE IS IT FROM?

Brown seaweeds are part of the *Phaeophyceae* class of algae, and grow underwater in cool, coastal regions. Wakame and kombu are the most commonly eaten varieties. Brown seaweeds are eaten fresh in their countries of origin, such as Japan, and are also dried or pickled.

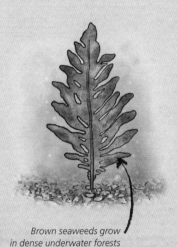

Brown seaweeds grow in dense underwater forests close to the coast

HOW TO EAT IT

1 VEGETABLE RAMEN

Kombu is a traditional addition to Japanese-style broths. Cook strips of dried kombu in stock, season with soy sauce, and add cooked noodles, cooked mixed vegetables, fried tofu, and a boiled egg for a simple, nutritious ramen bowl.

2 IN STIR-FRIES

Firm brown seaweeds, such as wakame, add texture and a rich, briny flavor to rice-based stir-fries. Add 1 tablespoon of soaked, drained, and chopped wakame to a brown rice power bowl (see pp32–33) for an instant flavor boost.

3 PICKLED KOMBU

Use pickled kombu to add flavor to rice dishes, as well as sandwiches and sushi wraps. Soak, rinse, and thinly slice 4–5 strips, then pickle for at least 1 hour in a rice vinegar and mirin solution.

TIP

Add kombu to bean-based soups and stews. The enzymes in kombu help predigest beans, reducing their flatulent effects.

Kombu is sold dried or pickled

The very large quantities of **iodine** in brown seaweed may help combat **fatigue**, **muscle weakness**, and high levels of **bad cholesterol**, as well as helping with **weight management**.

RED SEAWEED

Red seaweeds, including nori and dulse, are fiber-rich and low-fat, and contain many minerals, especially iodine, vital for thyroid function, and calcium, which promotes strong bones. Dulse is super-rich in potassium, nori in protein.

WHY EAT IT?

BLOOD HEALTH
Eating just a small amount of dulse fulfills your daily reference intake of the mineral potassium, which can help lower blood pressure by counteracting some of the negative effects of sodium.

HORMONE BALANCE
All seaweed is high in a group of phytoestrogens called lignans, which are believed to reduce the risk of breast cancer and help relieve some of the symptoms associated with PMS.

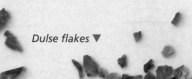

Dulse flakes ▼

HIGH IN IODINE

Red seaweeds are slightly lower in iodine than brown seaweeds, but are still an incredible source. Iodine is needed for a number of your body's processes, including growth, the regulation of the metabolism by the thyroid, and the development of a baby's brain during pregnancy and early life. An underactive thyroid can result in fatigue, muscle weakness, and high cholesterol levels.

Red seaweed, especially dulse, is rich in **potassium**, which has been shown to **lower blood pressure**.

WHAT'S IN IT?

A ⅓oz (10g) serving of nori is an excellent source of vitamin B12 and iodine, as well as vitamin A and potassium. Nori contains higher quantities of vitamins than dulse.

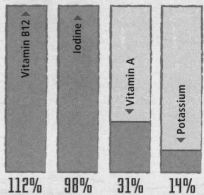

Vitamin B12	Iodine	Vitamin A	Potassium
112%	98%	31%	14%

Percentage of your daily reference intake

Nori sheets ▼

Dried dulse is available whole-leaf, flaked, or as a powder

Protein-rich nori turns black or green when dried

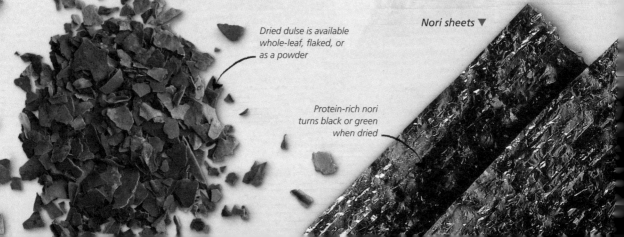

Red seaweed is a great source of the mineral **iodine**, which is important for the **regulation** of your **thyroid gland**, as well as helping in the development of a **baby's brain**.

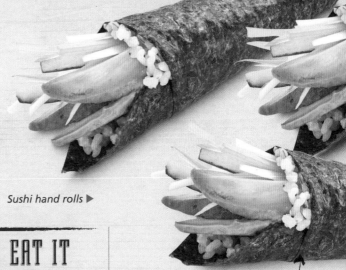

Sushi hand rolls ▶

WHERE IS IT FROM?

Red seaweeds owe their color to the pigment phycoerythrin. They include nori, which is cultivated in Japan, sold in sheets, and used to wrap sushi, and rich-flavored dulse, popular in Ireland and Scotland. Welsh laver and Irish moss also fall into this group of seaweeds.

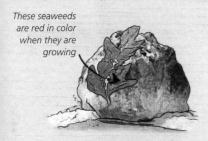

These seaweeds are red in color when they are growing

HOW TO EAT IT

1 SUSHI HAND ROLLS

Sushi rolling may be hard to master, but making a hand roll is far easier. Take cold, cooked whole-grain rice, lightly dressed with mirin, and roll up in a nori cone with avocado and cucumber sticks for a quick and healthy lunch.

2 SUPER SPRINKLE

Japanese rice dishes are often garnished with a sprinkle of furikake—a seaweed seasoning. Make your own by blending up dried nori, sesame seeds, red chile flakes, and sea salt to a coarse powder.

3 SEAWEED SALAD

This Asian-inspired seaweed salad is as healthy as it is addictive. Soak dried dulse briefly in water to reconstitute it, then dry and mix with shredded carrots and cucumber. Dress with a mixture of rice vinegar, sesame oil, ginger, and soy sauce.

Phytoestrogens in red seaweed may help **reduce** the risk of **breast cancer**.

Use fresh nori sheets so that they do not break when rolling

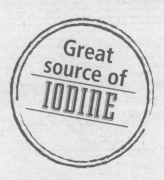

Great source of **IODINE**

TIP
If nori sheets kept in storage start to lose their crispness, toast them very carefully over the flame on a gas stove.

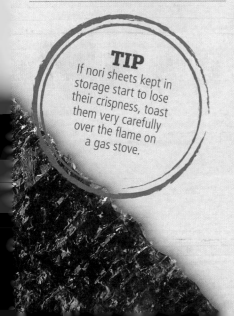

MAXIMIZE THE BENEFITS

KEEP NORI COOL AND DRY
Nori labeled as "plain" or "toasted" will keep well in a cool, dry place.

EAT FRESH OR DRIED DULSE
Fresh and dried dulse have similar levels of vitamins and other nutrients. Dried dulse can be used without soaking, in the form of whole leaves, flakes, or powder. Before using whole-leaf dulse, pull the fronds apart to remove any trapped pebbles.

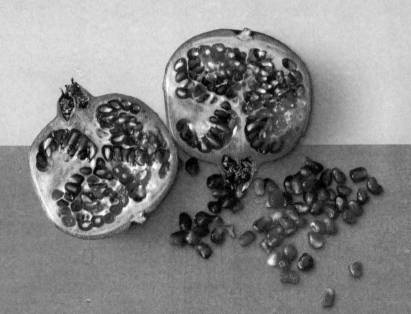

FRUIT

APPLES

A useful source of vitamins C, K, and B6, apples support your immune, skeletal, and circulatory systems. Phytochemicals in apples may keep your eyes healthy and help reduce bad cholesterol.

WHY EAT IT?

EYE HEALTH
Research suggests that quercetin—which is present in high quantities in apples—may help to protect against cataracts by inhibiting the damage from free radicals to your eyes.

DIGESTIVE HEALTH
Apples provide both soluble and insoluble fiber, which speed the passage of waste products through the digestive tract. Research from the University of Denmark found that people who regularly ate apples had high levels of "friendly" bacteria in their gut.

HEART HEALTH
Pectin, a type of soluble fiber found in apples, can help reduce high cholesterol levels. A study from Finland found that eating just one apple a day for 4 weeks reduced bad cholesterol by as much as 40 percent.

Apple skin contains fiber and vitamin C

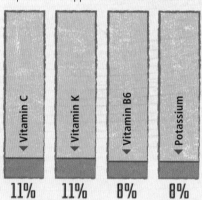

WHAT'S IN IT?

1 medium apple (5½oz/150g) is a useful source of vitamins C, K, and B6, as well as potassium. Apples also contain fiber.

Vitamin C	Vitamin K	Vitamin B6	Potassium
11%	11%	8%	8%

Percentage of your daily reference intake

WHERE IS IT FROM?

Apples are the fruits of a deciduous tree in the rose family. The apple tree is cultivated across the world, and exists in 7,000 varieties.

Apples grow from pale blossoms into red or green fruit

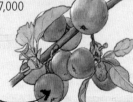

HOW TO EAT IT

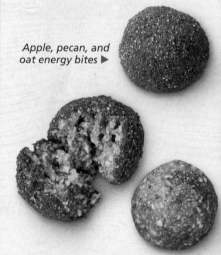

Apple, pecan, and oat energy bites ▶

1 APPLE, PECAN, AND OAT ENERGY BITES
Blend raw grated apple with dried fruit, nuts, and oats, and roll into balls to make nutritious snacks.

2 BAKED DESSERT
Core whole apples and stuff with a mixture of chopped nuts and dried fruit before baking until soft in a medium oven.

3 APPLE COLESLAW
Brighten up grilled fish or chicken with a quick 'slaw of apple, fennel, and white cabbage, dressed in lemon juice and olive oil.

FIGS

Both fresh and dried figs are rich in fiber and potassium, helping reduce bad cholesterol and keep your digestive and nervous systems healthy.

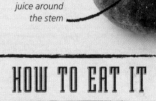

Ripe figs may have beads of natural sugar juice around the stem

WHY EAT IT?

DIGESTIVE HEALTH

Figs are a good source of both soluble and insoluble fiber, which helps to speed the passage of waste material through the digestive tract. The fruit can have a mild laxative effect. Dried figs contain more fiber than fresh: ⅓ cup of dried figs provides around 20 percent of the recommended daily amount of fiber. Figs also contain a type of fiber that helps to stimulate the growth of friendly bacteria in the colon.

HEART HEALTH

The soluble fiber in figs can help reduce high cholesterol in your blood. Figs also contain a group of phytochemicals called polyphenols that help protect your heart, and potassium, which can help lower high blood pressure.

BONE STRENGTH

Dried figs are a good source of calcium, making them a particularly useful food for people who don't consume dairy products. Calcium is vital for maintaining strong bones and teeth. Figs also contain vitamin K, which helps distribute calcium around your body and helps your bones absorb calcium.

WHAT'S IN IT?

2 fresh figs (3½oz/100g) provide a source of potassium, vitamin B6, calcium, and zinc. Figs also contain vitamins B1, B2, and K.

Potassium	Vitamin B6	Calcium	Zinc
10%	6%	5%	3%

Percentage of your daily reference intake

WHERE IS IT FROM?

Native to the Middle East and western Asia, figs are the fruits of a tree from the mulberry family that can live for up to 100 years.

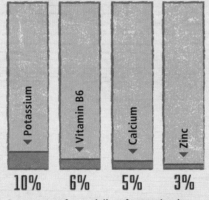

Different varieties are purple, green, or yellow in color

HOW TO EAT IT

1 **FIG CAKE**
For a sweet accompaniment to cheese and crackers, process dried figs with toasted almonds and a little honey, and press into a flat cake.

2 **EASY BAKE**
Sun-ripened figs are at their best simply baked. Drizzle with a little honey and bake until soft before serving warm with some Greek yogurt and chopped walnuts.

3 **STICKY JAM**
Pair sweet, sticky fig jam with the sharp flavors of goat cheese. Peel and cook down ripe figs to a thick paste and smear on crusty bruschetta with some soft cheese.

POMEGRANATE

Packed with vitamins B6 and C, fiber, and anthocyanins, pomegranates support your nerves, blood, brain, and immune system. They also contain antioxidants that may reduce the risk of heart disease and combat cancer.

WHY EAT IT?

HEART HEALTH

Pomegranates contain a group of phytochemicals called polyphenols—powerful antioxidants that are known to help reduce the risk of heart disease. Drinking pomegranate juice can help to reduce high blood pressure and improve blood flow to the heart.

CANCER PREVENTION

Antioxidants in pomegranates are believed to help protect cells and repair DNA damage that can lead to cancer. Some studies have found that pomegranate juice can help slow the growth of prostate cancer. Other research suggests that it may also help fight other types of cancer, including breast and colon cancer.

BRAIN POWER

Pomegranates get their distinctive color from phytochemicals called anthocyanins, which are believed to improve blood flow to the brain. Diets rich in anthocyanins are known to improve memory in later life.

Studies have shown that **pomegranate juice** may help **combat prostate, breast,** and **colon cancers**.

WHAT'S IN IT?

The seeds from 1 medium pomegranate (about 1 cup) provide a good source of vitamins B6 and C, as well as fiber and potassium.

Vitamin B6	Vitamin C	Fiber	Potassium
44%	32%	30%	24%

Percentage of your daily reference intake

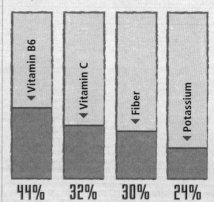

Pomegranate seeds are rich in fiber

Choose glossy fruits that feel heavy—these are likely to contain plenty of plump seeds

WHERE IS IT FROM?

Native to Iran, pomegranates are grown in Mediterranean-type climates around the world. The fruit is composed of cavities filled with many kernels. Each kernel consists of a small, crunchy or softish seed covered with brilliant ruby-red or white jelly.

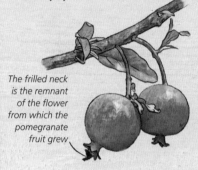

The frilled neck is the remnant of the flower from which the pomegranate fruit grew

HOW TO PREPARE

Cut off the top of the pomegranate. Score the skin into quarters, then break the fruit apart with your hands. Use your fingers or a spoon to remove the kernels from the fleshy membrane. Alternatively, halve the pomegranate and hit the back of it with a wooden spoon to knock the seeds out.

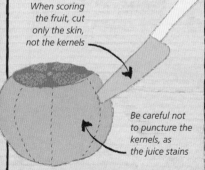

When scoring the fruit, cut only the skin, not the kernels

Be careful not to puncture the kernels, as the juice stains

HOW TO EAT IT

1 PURE JUICE
Blend or process the seeds to a purée, then press the resulting pulp through a fine strainer to release the juice. Sweeten with a little honey, as needed.

2 JEWELED JELLY
Set store-bought 100 percent pomegranate juice with some natural gelatin and scatter it with fresh pomegranate seeds to make a simple, elegant summer jelly.

3 TROPICAL FRUIT SALAD
Enjoy the vivid, jewel-like hue and natural crunch of pomegranate seeds in a fruit salad with chopped mango, pineapple, melon, and kiwi fruit.

Tropical fruit salad ▶

The **seeds** of **1 pomegranate** account for over **30 percent** of your daily **reference intake** of vitamin C.

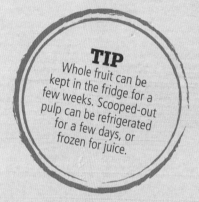

TIP
Whole fruit can be kept in the fridge for a few weeks. Scooped-out pulp can be refrigerated for a few days, or frozen for juice.

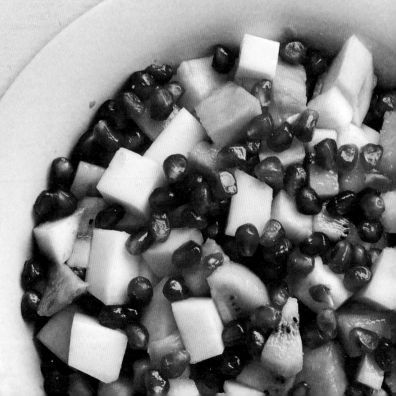

POMEGRANATE & RASPBERRY GRANITA

This fresh-tasting granita is a simple, superfood alternative to ice cream, and doesn't require an ice-cream maker. It's packed with antioxidant pomegranates, vitamin C—rich raspberries, and immune-boosting mint.

Serves 8 **Prep time** 15 minutes, plus freezing

INGREDIENTS

2¼lb (1kg) seedless watermelon (about 1½ mini-watermelons) or ½ large watermelon, rind removed and diced

1½ cups **raspberries**, plus extra to garnish

¾ cup **pomegranate** seeds, plus extra to garnish

large handful of **mint** leaves, plus extra to garnish

1–2 tbsp honey

SPECIAL EQUIPMENT

blender or food processor

2.6l (4½pt) freezer-proof lidded airtight container

METHOD

1 Place half the watermelon in the blender or food processor, along with half the raspberries, pomegranate seeds, and mint leaves. Process to a liquid and pour into a large bowl. Blend the remaining watermelon, raspberries, pomegranate seeds, and mint, and combine with the first batch of liquid. (Working in batches prevents the blender or food processor from overflowing.)

2 Pour the resulting liquid through a fine-mesh strainer into a large bowl, pressing down with the back of a spoon to extract all the liquid from the pulp. Discard the pulp. If you are using seeded watermelon, also discard any fragments of seed.

3 Whisk in the honey as needed, depending on the sweetness of the watermelon. Remember that the sweetness will be dulled on freezing, and adjust according to your taste.

4 Pour the liquid into the container and freeze. Remove from the freezer every 2 hours and use a metal fork to scrape the frozen sides back into the granita, crushing the resulting crystals as you go. Repeat three times, until it is completely frozen.

5 Remove from the freezer and put in the fridge for 30 minutes before serving. To serve, scrape out layers of crystals into individual serving bowls or glasses and garnish with extra raspberries, pomegranate seeds, and mint leaves.

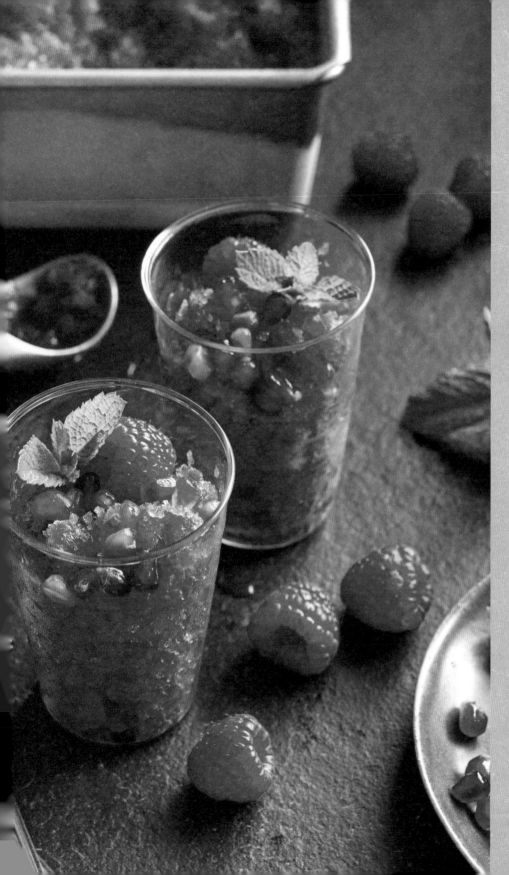

FEATURED SUPERFOODS

RASPBERRIES
help keep your **eyes** healthy

POMEGRANATE
may help fight certain
types of **cancer**

MINT
helps boost your
immune system

Nutrition
per serving

Energy 66cals (262kj)
Carbohydrate 13g
– of which sugars 13g
Fiber 2g
Fat 0g
– of which saturated 0g
Salt 0g
Protein 1g
Cholesterol 0g

PLUMS

Because plums are low GI, they satisfy a sweet tooth without causing spikes in blood sugar. They also provide heart-healthy potassium, antioxidant phytochemicals, and lots of gut-healthy fiber.

WHY EAT IT?

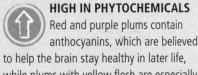

HIGH IN PHYTOCHEMICALS
Red and purple plums contain anthocyanins, which are believed to help the brain stay healthy in later life, while plums with yellow flesh are especially high in beta-carotene, which your body converts into vitamin A.

DIGESTIVE HEALTH
Plums and prunes (dried plums) are rich in fibers, such as pectin, as well as sorbitol and isatin, natural laxatives that help relieve constipation.

BONE STRENGTH
Emerging research suggests that eating prunes may help reduce the rate at which calcium is lost from the bones after menopause.

WHAT'S IN IT?

½ cup of sliced plums is a good source of potassium, vitamin K, copper, and vitamin A. Plums also contain fiber.

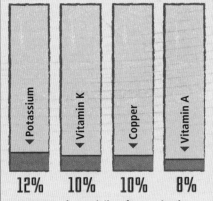

Potassium	Vitamin K	Copper	Vitamin A
12%	10%	10%	8%

Percentage of your daily reference intake

HOW TO EAT IT

1 BAKE THEM
Roast plum halves with honey, five spice, and star anise until soft. Serve with Greek yogurt for a healthy dessert.

2 PLUM GRANITA
Cook down pitted plums in a little water, honey, and spices. Purée, then put the resulting liquid through a fine-mesh strainer before freezing to make a simple yet elegant dark plum granita.

3 BARBECUE SAUCE
Cook plums with vinegar, honey, and spices, then purée until smooth and serve with barbecued meats.

WHERE IS IT FROM?

Related to cherries, plums are drupes, or stone fruits. There are several varieties originating from various temperate regions, including the Middle East, China, and the Americas.

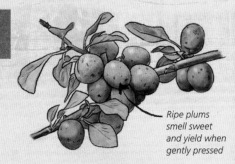

Ripe plums smell sweet and yield when gently pressed

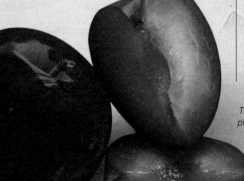

The skin contains different phytochemicals depending on its color

BLACK CURRANTS

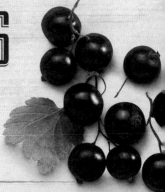

With off-the-scale levels of both anthocyanins and vitamin C, black currants offer a potent antioxidant boost to your immune system and heart health.

WHY EAT IT?

IMMUNE BOOST
Black currants are exceptionally rich in vitamin C (three times more than the same weight of oranges), which boosts the action of white blood cells.

HEART HEALTH
Rich in anthocyanins, black currants may help reduce the risk of heart disease and stroke.

DISEASE PREVENTION
The anthocyanins in black currants may help boost levels of friendly bacteria in the gut and reduce the risk of certain types of cancer. The high levels of vitamin C also help protect your body against infection.

Summer pudding ▼

WHAT'S IN IT?

A ¾-cup serving of fresh black currants is an excellent source of vitamin C, as well as potassium, manganese, and vitamin B6. Black currants also contain vitamins B1 and B2, as well as iron.

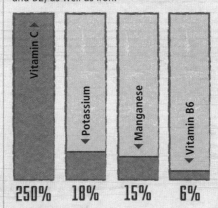

Vitamin C ▶	Potassium ▶	Manganese ▶	Vitamin B6 ▶
250%	**18%**	**15%**	**6%**

Percentage of your daily reference intake

WHERE IS IT FROM?

Black currants are the berries of a small shrub native to the northern hemisphere. The highly pigmented berries contain more antioxidants than currants of other colors.

Ripe berries are plump and dark purple in color

HOW TO EAT IT

1 RAW SUPERFOOD JAM
Blend fresh black currants with chia seeds, maple syrup, and lemon juice, and rest for 30 minutes to allow to thicken.

2 BREAKFAST PARFAIT
Lightly cook black currants with a little honey, then layer the resulting compote with Greek yogurt and granola.

3 SUMMER PUDDING
Spoon gently simmered black currants and other summer fruits, with their juices, into a basin lined with sliced white bread. Cover tightly, chill overnight, and turn the pudding out of the basin to serve.

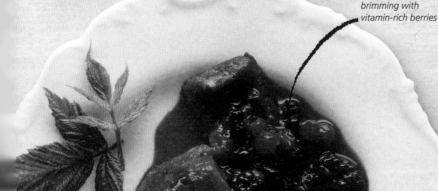

This dessert is brimming with vitamin-rich berries

EATING FOR SKIN HEALTH

The foods we eat are powerful tools for maintaining healthy skin and protecting it from sun damage and the effects of aging. Here is an example of a day of eating for skin health, incorporating the right foods into your diet in order to keep your skin glowing.

TO DRINK

Aim to drink 6–8 glasses of water, or other healthy fluids—such as herbal teas, tisanes, or coconut water—each day. Even mild dehydration causes your skin to look dry, gray, and tired. Drink before you feel thirsty, as a feeling of thirst is a sign that your body is already dehydrated.

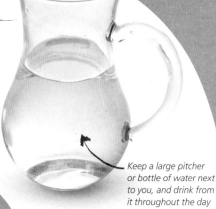

Keep a large pitcher or bottle of water next to you, and drink from it throughout the day

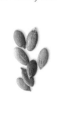

A large handful of pumpkin seeds provides almost a third of your daily reference intake of skin-healthy zinc

BREAKFAST

Make a vitamin C–rich smoothie of kiwi and apples—vitamin C acts as an antioxidant that helps prevent free radicals from causing wrinkling and other signs of skin aging. Pair this with a poached egg on whole-grain toast—this is low-GI and helps protect collagen, which prevents your skin from being damaged by high blood sugar.

MID-MORNING SNACK

Grab a handful of pumpkin seeds for a mid-morning snack. These seeds are rich in zinc, a vital mineral that supports the oil-producing glands in your skin and helps skin heal.

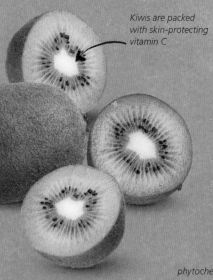

Kiwis are packed with skin-protecting vitamin C

Vitamins and phytochemicals in apples support skin health

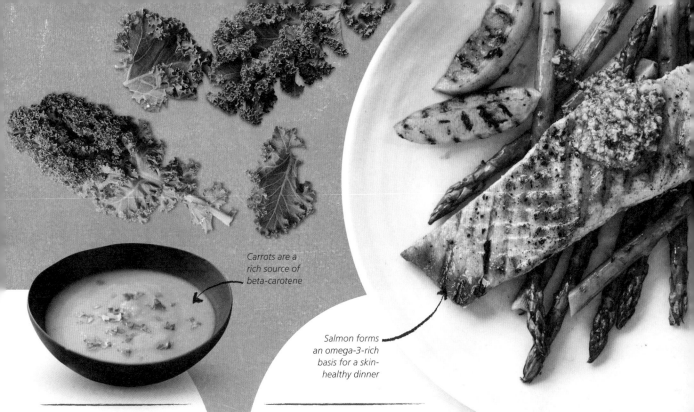

Carrots are a rich source of beta-carotene

Salmon forms an omega-3-rich basis for a skin-healthy dinner

LUNCH

Eat a simple carrot soup to support healthy skin. Beta-carotene is the phytochemical that lends carrots their bright color, and it can also help improve skin tone—it's converted into vitamin A in your body, which helps keep your skin glowing with health.

DINNER

The omega-3 fats found in salmon help your body to produce anti-inflammatory compounds, which help slow—and even reverse—signs of skin aging, as well as improving skin elasticity. Add a side dish of lightly cooked kale for a satisfying, skin-healthy dinner—kale contains the phytochemical lutein, which may help protect your skin against sun damage.

The lutein in kale may help protect your skin from sun damage

AFTERNOON SNACK

Rich in the antioxidant selenium, Brazil nuts can help protect skin against skin cancer, sun damage, and age spots. Eat a handful in the afternoon to tide you over until dinner.

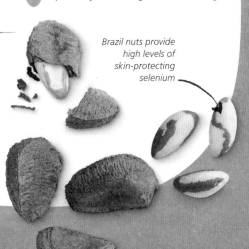

Brazil nuts provide high levels of skin-protecting selenium

EAT LOW-GI

High blood sugar levels may trigger a reaction in your skin called glycation, which damages the collagen that keeps your skin healthy and youthful looking. Choosing low-GI carbohydrates, such as whole grains, and avoiding sugary foods is the best way to avoid high blood sugar levels.

CHERRIES

Cherries earn their superfood status thanks to their high levels of phytochemicals, especially anthocyanins with antioxidant and anti-inflammatory properties, and melatonin, which can help regulate sleep.

WHY EAT IT?

HEALTHY SLEEP
Cherries contain the phytochemical melatonin, a hormone that helps regulate the body's internal clock and sleep-wake cycles. Studies have shown that drinking cherry juice can improve the quality and duration of sleep for people who suffer from insomnia.

HIGH IN ANTIOXIDANTS
Studies suggest that the antioxidants in cherries may act as an anti-inflammatory that helps to reduce pain from gout, arthritis, and muscular aches after exercise. They may also help protect against heart disease and certain cancers.

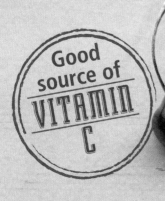

Good source of VITAMIN C

BRAIN POWER
Cherries get their ruby red color from phytochemicals known as anthocyanins. These antioxidant pigments have been shown to improve memory and cognitive function.

The phytochemical **melatonin** in cherries may help **improve** the **quality** and duration of your **sleep**.

Shiny skin and a bright green stem indicate freshness, and therefore more nutrients

WHAT'S IN IT?

A 1-cup serving of cherries provides useful quantities of vitamin C, potassium, copper, and vitamin B6. They also contain vitamins B1 and B2, as well as niacin.

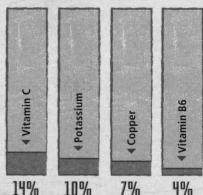

Vitamin C	Potassium	Copper	Vitamin B6
14%	10%	7%	4%

Percentage of your daily reference intake

WHERE IS IT FROM?

Native to Eastern Europe and Western Asia, cherries are the drupes, or stone fruits, of the cherry tree. The trees need sufficient winter cold to germinate and blossom, so they grow in temperate regions.

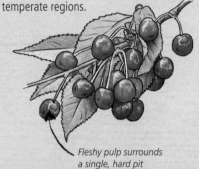

Fleshy pulp surrounds a single, hard pit

MAXIMIZE THE BENEFITS

EXTEND THE SEASON

When fresh cherries aren't in season, you can drink cherry juice or buy dried or frozen cherries. Both cherry juice and dried cherries contain similar levels of antioxidants to fresh cherries. Drying fruit increases its fiber content and can concentrate other nutrients, but reduces its vitamin C content and concentrates its natural sugars to higher levels.

HOW TO EAT IT

1 FROZEN TREATS

Instead of turning to chocolate or ice cream, try yogurt-coated frozen cherries as a sweet treat. Dip them in Greek yogurt flavored with vanilla extract, and freeze on a baking sheet for at least 30 minutes before serving.

2 PICKLED

Sweet–tart pickled cherries are wonderful served alongside cold meats and cheeses, or even in a sandwich. Pickle them in a spiced cider vinegar solution and store in a cool, dark place for at least 2 weeks before serving.

3 CHERRY COMPOTE

A glut of cherries can be put to use quickly and easily by making a compote. Cook down pitted cherries in a little water until they are soft and jamlike. Use the compote as a dessert, breakfast topping, or jam substitute.

Antioxidants are concentrated in the skin

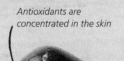

TIP

Cherries lose quality at room temperature, so store them in the fridge, unwashed, for 3–5 days. Freeze whole, or as pulp.

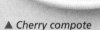

▲ *Cherry compote*

Cherries make a naturally sweet sauce without the need for added sugar

Research shows that **eating cherries** may help to **reduce** the risk of **heart disease** and certain types of **cancer**, due to their **high levels** of **antioxidants**.

BLUEBERRIES

Packed with antioxidants, blueberries help keep your heart and brain healthy. They are also a good source of the vital mineral manganese, which supports the circulatory and skeletal systems, and may help control blood sugar levels.

WHY EAT IT?

HEART HEALTH

The Iowa Women's Health Study monitored the diets of over 34,400 postmenopausal women over a period of 16 years. Researchers found that those women who ate blueberries at least once a week were significantly less likely to die from strokes or heart disease than those who didn't eat them.

Anti-inflammatory anthocyanin gives blueberries their deep, purple-blue color

BRAIN POWER

The antioxidants in blueberries are believed to protect your brain against signs of aging by increasing the flow of blood and oxygen to the brain. They also protect your brain from damage by free radicals that are believed to increase the risk of age-related memory loss, Alzheimer's disease, and dementia.

BLOOD HEALTH

Studies show that people who eat blueberries regularly are less likely to suffer from high blood pressure than those who don't. It is thought that the phytochemicals in blueberries help boost levels of nitric oxide, a chemical that helps relax and widen blood vessels, allowing blood to flow more freely.

Choose blueberries with a silvery bloom—these are fresh and rich in nutrients

WHAT'S IN IT?

¾ cup of fresh blueberries provides a good source of manganese, vitamins C and E, and copper. They also contain vitamins B1, B2, and B6, as well as niacin, folate, potassium, iron, and zinc.

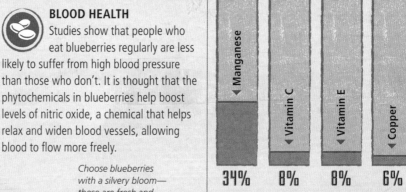

Manganese	Vitamin C	Vitamin E	Copper
34%	8%	8%	6%

Percentage of your daily reference intake

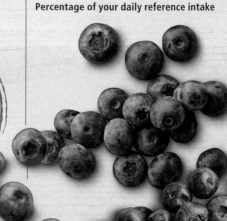

Good source of MANGANESE

MAXIMIZE THE BENEFITS

EAT FRESH AND DRIED

Fresh, frozen, and dried blueberries are all nutritionally beneficial. Dried blueberries contain the same levels of antioxidants as fresh and frozen berries, and more fiber—however, drying does destroy some of the vitamin C. Dried blueberries do not contain large quantities of added sugar, although natural sugars are concentrated during drying, so consume them in small quantities to avoid a spike in blood sugar.

WHERE IS IT FROM?

Native to the temperate woods and forests of the northern hemisphere, blueberries are the indigo-colored fruits of a flowering bush that is related to cranberries and bilberries. The berries were used as a coloring for cloth, baskets, and woodwork in precolonial and colonial North America.

Varieties with small berries tend to be more flavorful than varieties with large berries

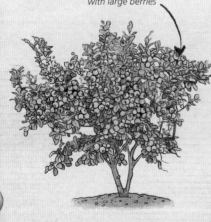

A large-scale study found that **regular consumption** of blueberries **reduced the risk** of **stroke** and **heart disease** for **older women**.

HOW TO EAT IT

1 FRUIT ROLL-UPS

Homemade fruit roll-ups, or fruit leather, is a naturally sweet treat that the whole family can enjoy. Purée blueberries with a little water, then spread thinly over a baking sheet and bake in a very low oven until dry.

2 QUICK COMPOTE

For a quick alternative to homemade jam, combine fresh blueberries with a little lemon juice and 1 teaspoon of maple syrup and cook until reduced to a syrupy texture. Enjoy hot or cold.

3 BLUEBERRY AND BANANA SMOOTHIE

Try using frozen blueberries for a chilled smoothie that's packed with antioxidants. Blend ½ cup of frozen blueberries with 2 tablespoons of yogurt, ⅓ cup of milk, and half of a banana.

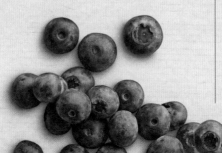

TIP
To freeze blueberries at home, spread them in a single layer on a large baking sheet before transferring to a freezer bag.

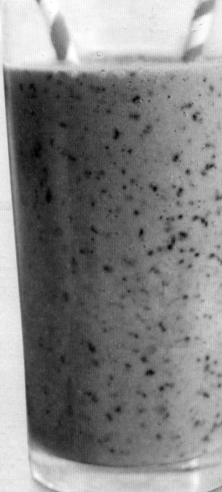

Blueberry and banana smoothie ▲

SUPER SMOOTHIE BOWL

Turn a simple smoothie into a nourishing breakfast bowl with the addition of antioxidant blueberries and raspberries, protein-rich nuts and seeds, and chia seeds, which are a useful source of omega-3 fats.

Serves 1   **Prep time** 5 minutes

INGREDIENTS

1/2 medium **papaya**, peeled, seeded, coarsely chopped, and frozen, about 2oz (60g) prepared weight

1 small **banana**, peeled, sliced, and frozen

1/2 cup **almond** milk

1 tbsp **almond** butter

2 tbsp Greek-style **yogurt**

honey (optional)

FOR THE TOPPING

fresh **blueberries**

fresh **raspberries**

homemade granola (see pp24–25)

sunflower seeds

chia seeds

sliced **almonds**

acai powder

SPECIAL EQUIPMENT

blender

METHOD

1 Simply place all the main ingredients in a blender and process until smooth and thick, adding a little extra almond milk if necessary.

2 Transfer the smoothie to a bowl and decorate with the superfood toppings. Sweeten the smoothie with a drizzle of honey, if needed.

SUPER SWAP

Replace the papaya, almond butter, and yogurt with apple, avocado, kale, and strawberries to benefit your skin, eyes, and bone health.

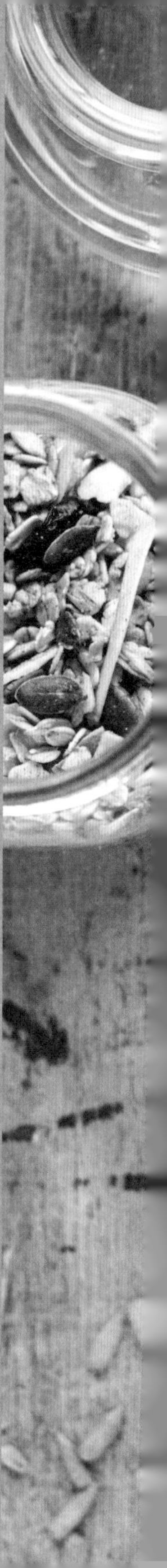

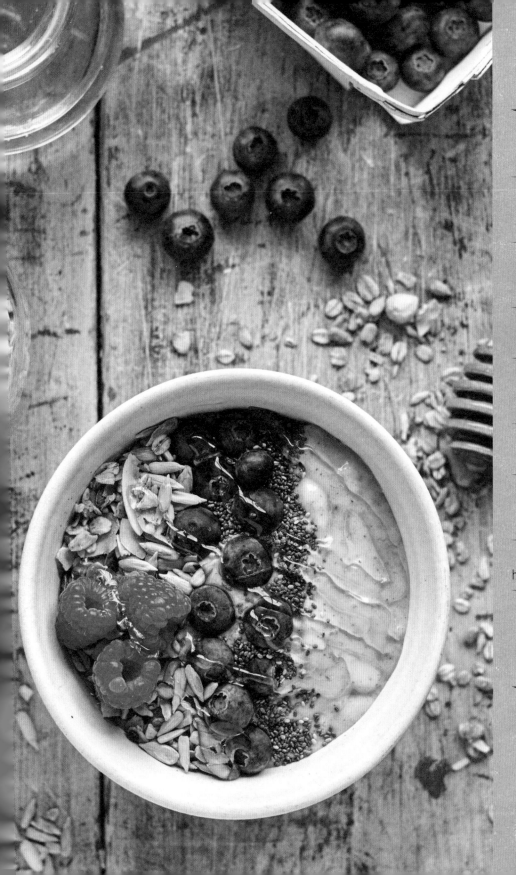

FEATURED SUPERFOODS

PAPAYA
helps maintain
digestive health

BANANA
may reduce high
blood pressure

ALMONDS
reduce the risk of
heart disease

YOGURT
helps maintain **gut health**

BLUEBERRIES
can help reduce the risk of
heart disease

RASPBERRIES
help keep your **eyes** healthy

SUNFLOWER SEEDS
help increase **good cholesterol**

CHIA SEEDS
help keep your **heart healthy**

ACAI POWER
can boost **energy levels**

Nutrition per serving

Energy 375cals (1530kj)
Carbohydrate 39g
– of which sugars 30g
Fiber 5.5g
Fat 20g
– of which saturated 10g
Salt 0.4g
Protein 6g
Cholesterol 37g

GOJI BERRIES

A rich source of copper and vitamin B2, goji berries may help boost your energy levels. They also contain a phytochemical that protects your eyes from damage.

WHY EAT IT?

EYE HEALTH
Goji berries get their vibrant red color from zeaxanthin, a phytochemical that is known to help protect the eyes from damage by free radicals.

ENERGY BALANCE
A study published in the *Journal of Alternative and Complementary Medicine* found that people who consumed goji berry juice for 14 days reported increased energy levels and mental alertness. Participants in the study also reported that they had improved quality of sleep.

IMMUNE BOOST
Early research suggests that goji berries, which are rich in antioxidants, may help strengthen the immune system and increase resistance to colds and flu.

Dried goji berries are richer in antioxidants than fresh goji berries

WHAT'S IN IT?

A 2-tablespoon serving of goji berries provides a good source of copper, vitamin B2, iron, and potassium. Goji berries also contain vitamins A and C.

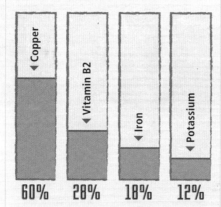

Copper	Vitamin B2	Iron	Potassium
60%	28%	18%	12%

Percentage of your daily reference intake

WHERE IS IT FROM?

Indigenous to the Himalayan mountain region of Tibet and China, goji berries are members of the nightshade family. They are also known as wolfberries.

HOW TO EAT IT

1 SUPER-SMOOTHIE POWDER
Dried goji berries can be hard to break down in a smoothie, but grind them first with some seeds, such as flaxseeds or chia seeds, and use the powder to enhance any smoothie.

2 REHYDRATE THEM
Soak dried goji berries in hot water for a few minutes, until soft and plump. Add to a rice or grain pilaf for a tomato-like zing.

3 BREAKFAST BARS
Decorate homemade cereal bars with a mixture of dried goji berries and pistachios for an eye-catching contrast.

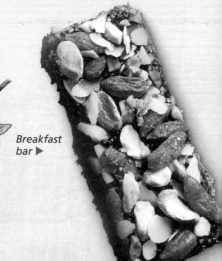

Breakfast bar ▶

CRANBERRIES

Cranberries are a good source of tissue- and bone-forming manganese, and contain antibacterial proanthocyanidins that help keep your stomach healthy.

WHY EAT IT?

IMMUNE BOOST
Drinking cranberry juice could help reduce the risk of recurrent urinary tract infections (UTIs), such as cystitis. Experts believe proanthocyanidins (PACs) in cranberries could prevent the bacteria that causes UTIs from sticking to the lining of the bladder and urinary tract.

DIGESTIVE HEALTH
The proanthocyanidins (PACs) present in cranberries may help protect against stomach ulcers. PACs prevent helicobacter pylori—bacteria that causes stomach ulcers—from attaching to your stomach lining.

HEART HEALTH
Some evidence suggests that the polyphenols in cranberries may reduce the risk of cardiovascular disease and reduce blood pressure.

Cranberries are best at their peak in winter, when shiny and red

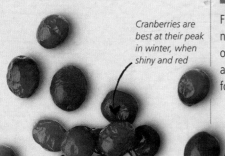

WHAT'S IN IT?

1 cup of cranberries provides a useful source of manganese, vitamin C, fiber, and vitamin B6. Cranberries also contain vitamins B, E, and K, as well as copper, zinc, iron, and potassium.

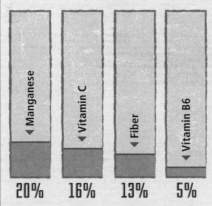

Manganese	Vitamin C	Fiber	Vitamin B6
20%	16%	13%	5%

Percentage of your daily reference intake

WHERE IS IT FROM?

Fruit of an evergreen shrub, cranberries are native to North America. Cranberries are often water-harvested, meaning that they are grown in wetlands and floated in water for easy harvesting.

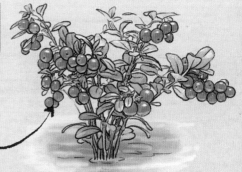

Ripe cranberries are firm, shiny, and bright red

HOW TO EAT IT

1 USE IN BAKING
Substitute dried cranberries for raisins or currants in any recipe to give your baked goods a superfood boost.

2 COMPOTE
Cranberry compote makes a great accompaniment to roast turkey. Cook fresh cranberries with a little fresh orange juice and zest until well-softened, then sweeten to taste with a little honey or maple syrup.

3 SUPER SALAD
Turn a simple green salad into a main meal rich with superfoods— add a handful each of dried cranberries, sliced almonds, and crumbled feta cheese.

WARM WINTER FRUIT COMPOTE

High in vitamin C and potassium, this warming compote supports your immune and nervous systems. Yogurt encourages the growth of good bacteria in your gut, and pistachios help maintain healthy cholesterol levels.

Serves 4   **Prep time** 15 minutes   **Cook time** 35 minutes

INGREDIENTS

3/4 cup dried apricots, coarsely chopped

3/4 cup dried prunes, coarsely chopped

1/4 cup dried **cherries**

1/2 cup dried **cranberries**

1 **cinnamon** stick

juice of 2 large **oranges**, plus the zest of 1

1 **apple**, peeled, cored, and coarsely chopped

1 pear, peeled, cored, and coarsely chopped

1/3 cup sliced **almonds**

Greek-style **yogurt**, to serve

chopped **pistachios**, to serve

METHOD

1 Place all the dried fruit in a medium, heavy-bottomed saucepan along with the cinnamon stick, orange juice and zest, and 1/2 cup of water.

2 Bring to a boil, then reduce to a low simmer and cook, covered, for 15 minutes.

3 Remove the lid and add the apple, pear, and almonds to the pan, carefully mixing them through the dried fruit. Cook for another 15 minutes, until the fresh fruit has softened.

4 Using a slotted spoon, remove the fruit from the pan and place in a heatproof bowl to cool. Discard the cinnamon stick and bring the cooking liquid back to a boil. Reduce to a simmer and cook, uncovered, for a few minutes until the liquid has reduced to a thick, dark syrup.

5 Pour the warm syrup over the cooked fruit and serve immediately, with Greek-style yogurt and chopped pistachios on top.

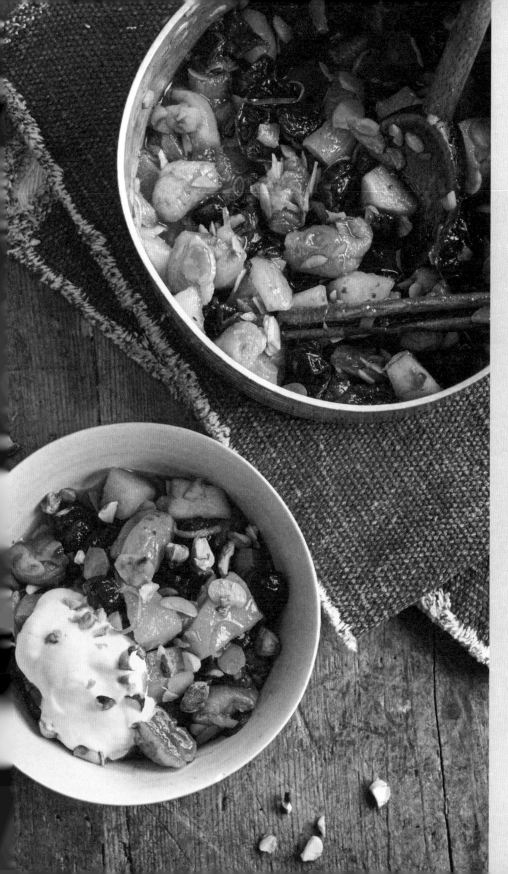

FEATURED SUPERFOODS

CHERRIES
may improve your **memory recall**

CRANBERRIES
prevent recurrent **urinary tract infections**

CINNAMON
helps **lower blood sugar levels**

ORANGES
support your **immune system**

APPLES
may help **protect eyes** from damage by free radicals

ALMONDS
reduce the risk of **heart disease**

YOGURT
helps maintain **gut health**

PISTACHIOS
help balance **cholesterol**

Nutrition per serving

Energy 268cals (1069kj)
Carbohydrate 47g
– of which sugars 46g
Fiber 7.5g
Fat 5g
– of which saturated 0.5g
Salt 0g
Protein 5g
Cholesterol 0g

STRAWBERRIES

Strawberries contain more vitamin C than oranges, and are rich in the B vitamin folate, energy-boosting manganese, and potassium, which supports heart health.

WHY EAT IT?

BLOOD HEALTH
Strawberries are rich in the B vitamin folate, which is important for the production of red blood cells. A good intake of folate is also important in the first 12 weeks of pregnancy, because it helps reduce the risk of birth defects such as spina bifida.

SKIN HEALTH
Strawberries contain ellagic acid, an antioxidant phytochemical that protects your skin from the damaging effects of sunlight and reduces the breakdown of collagen.

EYE HEALTH
A study published in the *Archives of Ophthalmology* suggests that eating three or more portions of strawberries, which are rich in vitamin C, may reduce the risk of age-related macular degeneration (AMD) by 36 percent.

Antioxidant flavonoids give strawberries their bright hue

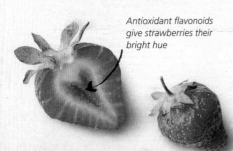

WHAT'S IN IT?

A ¾-cup serving of fresh strawberries provides a good source of vitamin C, folate, manganese, and potassium.

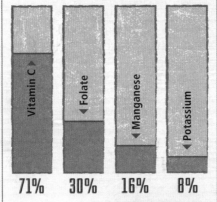

Vitamin C	Folate	Manganese	Potassium
71%	30%	16%	8%

Percentage of your daily reference intake

WHERE IS IT FROM?

Part of the rose family, strawberry plants are grown in temperate regions across the world. Now ubiquitous, garden strawberries were first developed in Europe during the 1700s.

Ripe berries are uniformly bright red in color

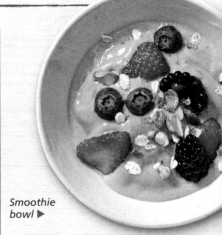

Smoothie bowl ▶

HOW TO EAT IT

1 SMOOTHIE BOWL
When you need something more substantial than a smoothie, try a smoothie bowl. Loaded with fruits, nuts, and seeds, it becomes a meal in its own right.

2 ADD TO A SALAD
Try adding fresh strawberries to a baby spinach salad, along with crumbled goat cheese and a balsamic vinaigrette.

3 STRAWBERRY ICE POPS
Making your own ice pops is super simple. Purée very ripe, sweet strawberries. Pour the purée into molds and freeze for at least 3 hours, until set.

RASPBERRIES

Packed with phytochemicals and vitamin C, raspberries support your skin and eye health. They also contain manganese, which helps your body produce energy.

WHY EAT IT?

EYE HEALTH
Raspberries contain lutein and vitamin C. Together they help protect the eyes from free radicals that increase the risk of cataracts and age-related macular degeneration (AMD).

SKIN HEALTH
The antioxidant phytochemical ellagic acid helps protect your skin from sunlight and reduces the breakdown of collagen.

ENERGY BALANCE
Raspberries have a low glycemic index (GI), which means they release sugar into your bloodstream more slowly compared to many other fruits, avoiding spikes in blood sugar.

TIP
Choose frozen raspberries or recently harvested fresh raspberries, as these contain similar levels of antioxidants.

WHAT'S IN IT?

A ¾-cup serving of fresh raspberries provides a good source of vitamin C, manganese, folate, and copper.

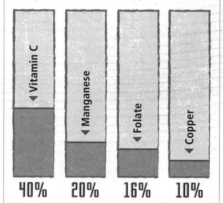

Vitamin C	Manganese	Folate	Copper
40%	20%	16%	10%

Percentage of your daily reference intake

WHERE IS IT FROM?

Native to eastern Asia, the raspberry plant is related to the rose family. They are widely grown in temperate regions and are found in a variety of colors.

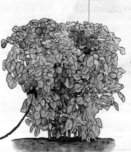

Raspberry fruits are harvested when they have turned a deep color

HOW TO EAT IT

1 RASPBERRY COULIS
A quick raspberry coulis can turn a simple dessert into something special. Cook fresh or frozen raspberries down slowly, strain to remove the seeds, and sweeten to taste with a little honey.

2 FRUITY GRANITA
Use fresh or frozen raspberries, puréed and strained, to make a granita (see pp146–47).

3 FREEZE-DRIED
Freeze-dried raspberries are increasingly easy to find, and are a rich source of antioxidants. Their bright color and sharp, zingy flavor is a welcome addition to any breakfast bowl or smoothie.

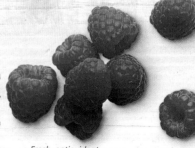

Fresh, antioxidant-rich berries should be firm and dry

BANANAS

Containing starch and fiber, bananas are an excellent superfood for your digestive health. They are a good source of heart-healthy potassium, as well as amino acids and vitamin B6, which help keep your brain healthy.

HEART HEALTH

Bananas are a good source of the mineral potassium. A diet rich in potassium counterbalances some of the negative effects of sodium, helping reduce high blood pressure and keep your heart healthy. Surveys show that many of us do not consume enough potassium, but people who eat high-potassium diets have been shown to live longer lives and be up to 24 percent less likely to have a stroke.

DIGESTIVE HEALTH

A rich source of fiber and resistant starch—a type of starch that doesn't break down in your intestines—bananas speed the passage of waste through the digestive system. Bananas also contain fructooligosaccharides (FOS), a type soluble fiber that encourages the growth of healthy bacteria in your gut.

BRAIN POWER

Bananas contain the amino acid tryptophan, which encourages the brain to produce serotonin, the "feel-good" hormone. They are also a good source of vitamin B6, which helps your body manufacture neurotransmitters—the chemicals that send messages between cells in your brain.

1 medium banana (3½oz/100g) is a good source of vitamin B6, manganese, potassium, and vitamin B1. Bananas also contain vitamins C and B2.

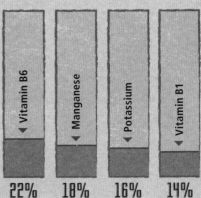

Vitamin B6	Manganese	Potassium	Vitamin B1
22%	18%	16%	14%

Percentage of your daily reference intake

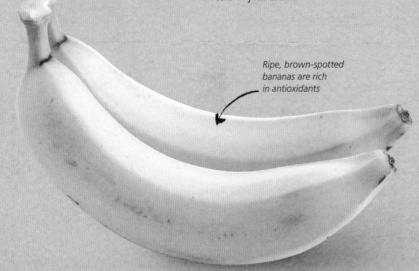

Ripe, brown-spotted bananas are rich in antioxidants

Bananas are a good source of **potassium**. People with diets **high** in potassium are up to **24 percent** less likely to have a **stroke**.

MAXIMIZE THE BENEFITS

EAT RIPE AND UNRIPE

Unripe bananas with green-tinged skin contain the highest levels of resistant starch, which helps speed the passage of waste material through your stomach and small intestine. As bananas ripen, the starch turns to sugar, but antioxidant levels increase. To consume bananas when they contain the highest levels of skin- and eye-protecting antioxidants, wait until the skin is yellow with a few brown or black spots.

WHERE IS IT FROM?

Grown throughout the tropics, the banana plant was first domesticated in the Wahgi Valley, Papua New Guinea, around 8000 BCE. Botanically, the plant is classified as an herb—the world's largest herb—rather than a tree. Each plant bears just one large bunch of bananas, separated into clusters of between 10 and 20 fruit, and must be pruned back after each harvest in order to fruit again.

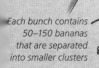

Each bunch contains 50–150 bananas that are separated into smaller clusters

HOW TO EAT IT

1 FRUIT-BASED SMOOTHIE

Bananas are the foundation of most fruit-based smoothies—they add bulk and reduce down to a thick, creamy texture once blended. Try mixing with overnight-soaked oats, almond milk, and maple syrup for a filling breakfast drink.

2 DAIRY-FREE ICE CREAM

Frozen bananas make a delicious dairy-free ice cream, with no need for added fat or sugar. Simply freeze chunks of banana, and then blend with a little vanilla extract until smooth. Refreeze for 10 minutes to firm up, if necessary.

3 CHIA AND BANANA BOWL

Turn an overnight chia pudding (see pp64–65) into a hearty breakfast with the addition of sliced banana, granola, and strawberries. Top it with seeds and cacao nibs for extra flavor and nutrients.

Chia and banana bowl ▶

The **soluble fiber** in bananas encourages the growth of **gut-friendly bacteria**, helping keep your **digestive system** healthy.

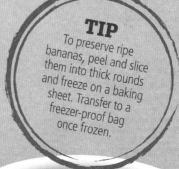

TIP

To preserve ripe bananas, peel and slice them into thick rounds and freeze on a baking sheet. Transfer to a freezer-proof bag once frozen.

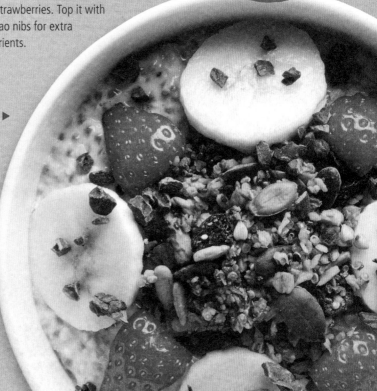

PINEAPPLE

Pineapple is a good source of immune-boosting vitamin C and a unique enzyme called bromelain, which supports your skeletal, digestive, and circulatory systems.

WHY EAT IT?

BONE AND JOINT HEALTH
Pineapple contains an enzyme called bromelain, which can help reduce inflammation and pain associated with arthritis.

DIGESTIVE HEALTH
The bromelain in pineapple helps break down protein in food, making it easier to digest. Pineapples are also a useful source of gut-healthy fiber.

BLOOD HEALTH
Research suggests that the bromelain in pineapple may reduce the stickiness of blood, making it useful for people at high risk of blood clots.

Juicy pineapple chunks are good for heart, digestion, and joints

WHAT'S IN IT?

½ cup of fresh pineapple is a good source of vitamin C, manganese, copper, and potassium. It also contains vitamins B1, B2, and B6, as well as fiber.

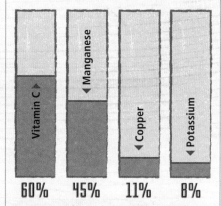

Vitamin C	Manganese	Copper	Potassium
60%	45%	11%	8%

Percentage of your daily reference intake

WHERE IS IT FROM?

The pineapple plant originates in the Americas, and is cultivated in tropical regions. Flowers fuse together to form a fruit at the heart of the plant.

Each large fruit sits amid spiked leaves

HOW TO EAT IT

1 AS A COOL DRINK
If you have a leftover half a pineapple, peel, chop, and freeze it. Blend the frozen pineapple chunks with a little apple juice for an instant frozen slushie.

2 DEHYDRATE IT
Dry thin slices of pineapple in a very low oven for a super-sweet fruity snack or addition to homemade granola.

3 PINEAPPLE SKEWERS
For a simple summer dessert, brush pineapple chunks with a little honey and grill on a barbecue until well-marked.

Pineapple skewers ▶

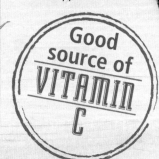

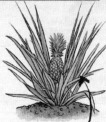

Good source of **VITAMIN C**

COCONUT

Its high fat content makes it a controversial superfood, but coconut is a rich source of fiber and energy-boosting manganese. The plant also produces a low-GI sweetener.

WHY EAT IT?

DIGESTIVE HEALTH
A good source of fiber, coconut flesh helps keep your digestive system healthy.

HIGH IN MANGANESE
Coconut is a useful source of manganese, which is needed for chemical processes in your body, including energy production. This mineral helps keep the blood, brain, and nerves healthy. Studies have linked low levels of manganese with an increased risk of osteoporosis.

ENERGY BALANCE
Coconut sugar has a low glycemic index (GI), providing slow-release energy for your body.

WHAT'S IN IT?

1 cup of fresh shredded coconut is a good source of manganese, copper, potassium, and phosphorus. Fresh coconut also contains vitamins B6, C, and E, as well as folate, magnesium, iron, zinc, selenium, iodine, and fiber.

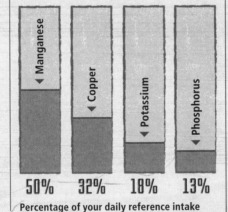

Manganese	Copper	Potassium	Phosphorus
50%	32%	18%	13%

Percentage of your daily reference intake

WHERE IS IT FROM?

Coconut palms grow in tropical regions close to the seashore. The flowers are harvested and processed into coconut sugar, or left to mature into hard-shelled fruit.

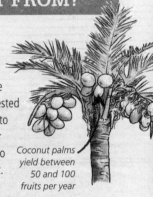

Coconut palms yield between 50 and 100 fruits per year

HOW TO EAT IT

1 IN ICE POPS
Make a dairy-free treat by blending coconut flesh with fresh mango and a squeeze of lime, and freezing until solid.

2 COCONUT 'SLAW
Make a bright, zingy Asian 'slaw using shredded fresh coconut, apple, and celeriac. Dress with a chile and lime vinaigrette for a flavorful side dish.

3 FOR BREAKFAST
Add dried coconut flakes to your morning granola or muesli, or use them to top a bowl of oatmeal or chia pudding.

Fiber-rich coconut flesh sits inside a hairy shell

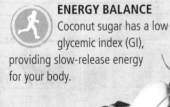

ORANGES

All citrus fruits contain high levels of vitamins, but oranges are supreme thanks to their abundance of vitamin C, flavonoids such as hesperetin, and other antioxidants and nutrients, which protect the heart and immune system.

WHY EAT IT?

HIGH IN VITAMIN C

A powerful antioxidant that helps keep skin youthful by neutralizing free radicals that accelerate wrinkling, vitamin C also strengthens the immune system and reduces the risk of cataracts, dementia, and some cancers.

BRAIN POWER

Oranges contain bioflavonoids (a group of phytochemicals), including hesperetin, thought to reduce age-related memory loss. Also, research shows that women consuming two or more servings of citrus fruits per day have an 18 percent lower risk of depression than those eating less than one serving weekly.

HEART HEALTH

Studies show that people who eat citrus fruit, such as oranges, regularly have a lower risk of heart disease and stroke. Phytochemicals in citrus are believed to improve the elasticity of the blood vessels, which improves flow of blood through the coronary arteries.

The **vitamin C** in oranges, a powerful **antioxidant**, helps to keep skin looking younger by neutralizing the **free radicals** that accelerate wrinkling.

WHAT'S IN IT?

1 medium orange (5¼oz/150g) provides high quantities of vitamin C and a good amount of vitamin B1, as well as folate and potassium. Oranges also contain vitamins A, B2, B6, and E, as well as niacin, phosphorus, magnesium, and copper.

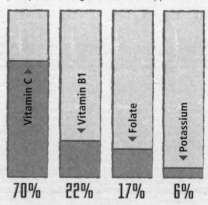

Vitamin C	Vitamin B1	Folate	Potassium
70%	22%	17%	6%

Percentage of your daily reference intake

Orange flesh is rich in pectin, a form of fiber that helps reduce bad cholesterol

Oranges and other citrus fruits lower the risk of **heart disease** and **stroke**, owing to **antioxidants** and **potassium**, which are good for blood flow.

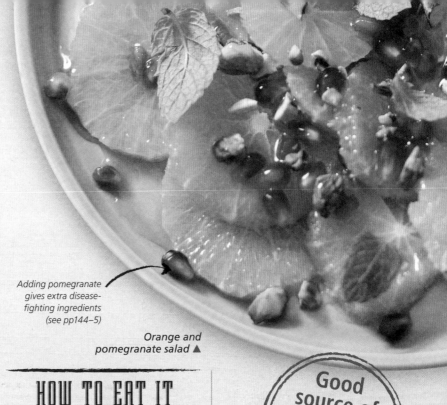

Adding pomegranate gives extra disease-fighting ingredients (see pp144–5)

Orange and pomegranate salad ▲

(see pp144–5)

WHERE IS IT FROM?

The orange is a citrus commercially grown in Mediterranean and subtropical regions worldwide, especially in Spain, the U.S., Brazil, China, and Mexico. There are many varieties, with different characteristics including size, thickness of skin, and flavor (from sharp to sweet). The world's leading commercial variety of orange is the Spanish Valencia. Mandarins are smaller and flatter, and less acid in flavor; within the mandarin group are tangerines and clementines.

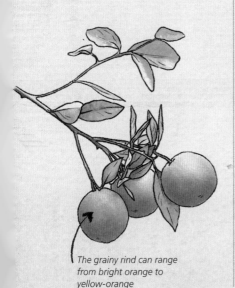

The grainy rind can range from bright orange to yellow-orange

HOW TO EAT IT

1 ORANGE AND POMEGRANATE SALAD
Oranges are often thought of as sweet, but they complement savory dishes, too. Try matching a simple salad of oranges, pomegranate, mint leaves, and pistachios with grilled fish or rosemary chicken skewers.

2 IN A SOUP
Freshly squeezed orange juice gives a bright, zesty boost to naturally sweet vegetables. Add finely chopped rosemary and the juice of a squeezed orange to homemade carrot or pumpkin soup.

3 BROILED ORANGES
A plate of broiled oranges makes a healthy, colorful breakfast offering. Simply mix 1 teaspoon of honey with spices such as ground cinnamon and allspice, coat onto the oranges, and then broil under high heat until golden brown.

Good source of VITAMIN C

MAXIMIZE THE BENEFITS

FAVOR THE WHOLE FRUIT
For snacking or breakfast, whole fruit is a healthier option than juice, since it is richer in antioxidants and fiber.

OPT FOR FRESHNESS
Buy fresh fruits that feel firm: the peels should yield to gentle pressure but bounce immediately. Fresh oranges should feel heavy for their size and have a sweet aroma. Avoid any oversoft oranges with spots or mold, as they will perish quicker.

BLOOD ORANGE & BEET SALAD

This sweet, crunchy salad is high in potassium and vitamin C from the oranges and beets, helping keep your blood and immune system healthy. Raw fennel contains phytochemicals that stimulate your digestive tract.

Serves 4   **Prep time** 20 minutes   **Cook time** 30 minutes, plus cooling

INGREDIENTS

2 medium-sized
   beets, peeled

1 tbsp olive oil

salt and freshly ground
   black pepper

¼ cup **walnuts**,
   coarsely chopped

2 small blood **oranges**

1 small **fennel** bulb, trimmed

2 cups **watercress**,
   washed and dried

3½ cups baby arugula,
   washed and dried

FOR THE DRESSING

¼ cup extra-virgin olive oil

1 tsp Dijon **mustard**

salt and freshly ground
   black pepper

METHOD

1 Preheat the oven to 400°F (200°C). Cut the beets into thin wedges, about 8 pieces per beet, and toss in the olive oil. Season well with salt and pepper, then roast for 30 minutes, turning once, until they are softened and charred at the edges. Set aside to cool.

2 Dry-fry the walnut pieces for 2–3 minutes over medium heat, stirring constantly, until browned in places. Set aside to cool.

3 Prepare the oranges by peeling with a small, sharp knife, being careful to remove all the white pith. Use the knife to cut out each segment, leaving the dividing pith behind. Squeeze all the remaining juice out of the leftover orange "skeleton" into a bowl. Repeat with the second orange, setting the segments aside.

4 To make the dressing, add the extra-virgin olive oil, Dijon mustard, and seasoning to the extracted orange juice, and whisk well to combine. Slice the fennel very finely and toss it in the dressing immediately, to keep it from discoloring.

5 Toss the prepared salad leaves with the fennel and dressing, then place on a large serving platter and top with the roasted beets, blood orange segments, and toasted walnuts. Serve immediately.

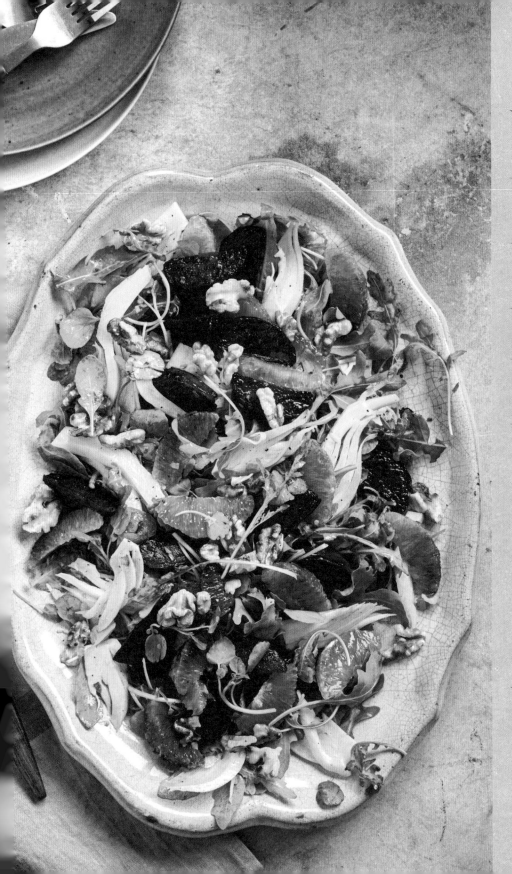

FEATURED SUPERFOODS

BEETS
may help maintain
heart health

WALNUTS
may help boost your
immune system

ORANGES
support your
immune system

FENNEL
may aid **digestion**

WATERCRESS
may help prevent certain
types of **cancer**

MUSTARD
is **anti-inflammatory**
and **antioxidant**

Nutrition per serving

Energy 228cals (908kj)

Carbohydrate 7.5g
– of which sugars 7g

Fiber 3.5g

Fat 19.5g
– of which saturated 2.5g

Salt 0.2g

Protein 4g

Cholesterol 0g

LEMONS

A rich source of phytochemicals and vitamin C, lemons help boost your immune system and neutralize free radicals that cause disease and skin aging. Lemons also protect against heart disease and help improve blood flow to your brain.

WHY EAT IT?

HIGH IN VITAMIN C
The high levels of vitamin C in lemons support your body in a number of ways. Vitamin C protects the cells that make up your immune system and boosts the action of bacteria- and virus-combating white blood cells. It also helps neutralize free radicals that are linked with heart disease, cancer, skin aging, and an increased risk of cataracts.

HEART HEALTH
Lemons are a rich source of a group of phytochemicals called bioflavonoids, which have been shown to help prevent heart disease. Studies show that women who eat citrus fruits regularly have a 19 percent lower risk of heart disease compared with those who don't eat them.

BRAIN POWER
Hesperetin, naringin, and naringenin are phytochemicals found in lemons that are believed to help improve blood flow to your brain, reducing the risk of age-related memory loss.

Women who eat citrus fruits regularly have a **19 percent lower** risk of **heart disease** than women who don't.

WHAT'S IN IT?

The juice of 1 medium lemon (3½oz/100g) provides a good source of vitamin C, copper, vitamin B6, and potassium. Lemons also contain vitamins B1 and B2.

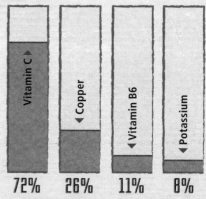

Vitamin C	Copper	Vitamin B6	Potassium
72%	26%	11%	8%

Percentage of your daily reference intake

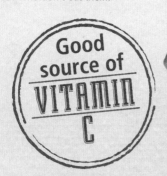

Good source of VITAMIN C

The peel is particularly rich in immune-boosting vitamin C

WHERE IS IT FROM?

Lemons are the fruit of a small tree in the *Rutaceae* family. The lemon tree is thought to originate in Oceania or Southeast Asia, and was brought to Spain and northern Africa around 1000–1200 CE. Today, lemons are cultivated in Mediterranean-type climates worldwide. The tree grows to around 20ft (6m) in height, and begins to bear fruit after about 3 years.

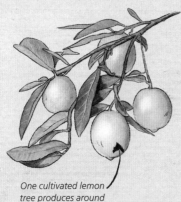

One cultivated lemon tree produces around 1,500 lemons each year

MAXIMIZE THE BENEFITS

SQUEEZE FRESH
Choose fresh, organic lemons for maximum nutrients. Squeeze your lemon juice just before you use it, and add in at the end of cooking to preserve nutrients.

EAT THE PEEL
Lemon peel contains higher quantities of vitamin C than lemon juice, but can taste bitter. Use the peel of organic lemons, and incorporate it into recipes in the form of zest or preserved lemons.

HOW TO EAT IT

1 IN LEMONADE
Make your own lemonade for a vitamin C boost with minimal added sugar. Mix freshly squeezed lemon juice with a little honey, then combine with sparkling water. Taste and add extra honey, if necessary.

2 PRESERVED LEMONS
Wash and slice organic lemons. Remove any seeds, and pack into a sterilized jar with plenty of sea salt and woody herbs, such as thyme or rosemary. Press each layer down to release the juices. Store at room temperature for 2 weeks before adding to salads or Moroccan-style stews, or serving with grilled fish.

3 LEMON SORBET
Sorbets are a way of indulging in a frozen treat without the addition of cream and sugar. Combine 1¼ cups of lemon juice with the same quantity of water, sweeten with honey to taste, and churn in an ice-cream maker for 30–40 minutes.

Lemon sorbet ▶

Phytochemicals found in lemons may **reduce** the **risk** of **memory loss** in old age by **improving blood flow** to the **brain**.

TIP
Store whole fruit in the fridge for up to 2 weeks. Allow to come to room temperature before using, as this will yield more juice.

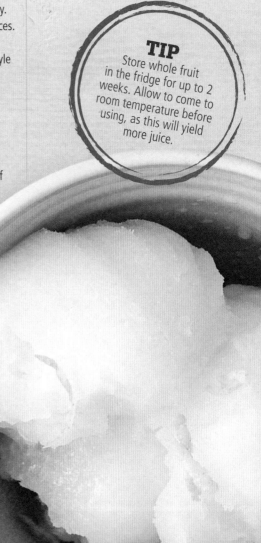

GUAVAS

Exceptional levels of vitamin C give guavas superfood status, but they have many other nutrients, too, including folate, which supports blood health.

WHY EAT IT?

IMMUNE BOOST
Weight for weight, guavas have four times more immunity-enhancing vitamin C than oranges.

DISEASE PREVENTION
Guavas contain several phytochemicals, including lycopene and quercetin, that have been shown to help reduce the risk of heart disease and certain types of cancer.

EYE HEALTH
The high levels of vitamin C in guavas may help reduce the risk of cataracts. Guavas are also a useful source of vitamin A, important for healthy eyes.

WHAT'S IN IT?

A ½-cup serving of sliced guava is an excellent source of vitamin C, and a good source of folate, copper, and potassium. Guava also contains vitamins A, E, B1, B2, and B6, as well as niacin, magnesium, manganese, and fiber.

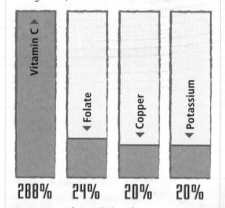

Vitamin C	Folate	Copper	Potassium
288%	24%	20%	20%

Percentage of your daily reference intake

HOW TO EAT IT

1 ADD TO VINAIGRETTE
Use the freshly pressed juice of a ripe guava as the base of a simple vinaigrette to dress baby spinach or a mixed-leaf salad.

2 GUAVA JUICE
Guava juice has a beautiful pink color. Use a juicer to extract the maximum amount of juice from the flesh, and serve with ice and mint for a cooling summer drink.

3 IN CHUTNEY
Guava chutney is a popular dish in South India to serve alongside snacks or flatbreads. Cook 1lb 2oz (500g) guava down to a soft consistency with spices and a little honey and vinegar.

WHERE IS IT FROM?

Guava, which thrives in tropical and subtropical regions, is an evergreen shrub or small tree that is thought to have originated in Central America. In non-tropical climates it is deciduous. The round fruits grow up to 3in (7.5cm) in diameter.

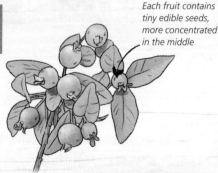

Each fruit contains tiny edible seeds, more concentrated in the middle

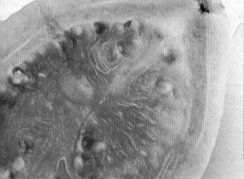

PAPAYAS

Papayas are a rich source of phytochemicals and vitamins C and A, helping support eye health and protect against disease.

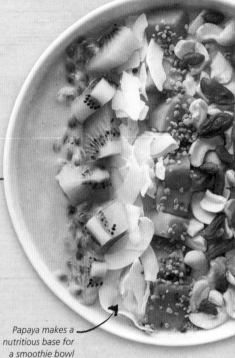

Papaya makes a nutritious base for a smoothie bowl

Papaya smoothie bowl ▲

WHY EAT IT?

EYE HEALTH
Papayas contain zeaxanthin, a phytochemical that protects the retina and lens of the eye from damage by free radicals and helps reduce the risk of age-related macular degeneration (AMD). Vitamins C and A found in papayas are also important for eye health.

DIGESTIVE HEALTH
Papayas contain an enzyme called papain, which can help break down protein and aid digestion. Papaya also offers good amounts of fiber.

DISEASE PREVENTION
The beta-carotene found in papayas may help lower the risk of certain types of cancer.

Scoop out and discard the dark-colored seeds

WHAT'S IN IT?

A ¾-cup serving of cubed papaya is rich in vitamin C, with good levels of vitamin A, folate, and potassium. Papaya also contains vitamins B1 and B2.

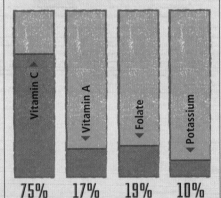

Vitamin C	Vitamin A	Folate	Potassium
75%	17%	19%	10%

Percentage of your daily reference intake

WHERE IS IT FROM?

Also called pawpaw, papaya grows in tropical or sub-tropical regions, such as Hawaii and South Africa.

Both ripe, yellow fruits and unripe, green fruits can be eaten

HOW TO EAT IT

1 PAPAYA SMOOTHIE BOWL
Papayas blend well to a thick, smooth texture and make a great base for a smoothie bowl, topped with more tropical fruits, such as kiwi and guava.

2 WITH LIME JUICE
Papayas are sometimes described as having a slightly musty taste. However, the sharp taste of lime juice transforms their flavor—try them with a squeeze of lime and a little chile pepper and salt.

3 GREEN PAPAYA SALAD
Green papayas are used to make one of the most popular Thai salads—Som Tam. They are mixed with shredded vegetables and dressed with crushed peanuts and a sweet-and-sour dressing.

MATCHA PANNA COTTA WITH TROPICAL FRUIT

This dairy-free panna cotta is flavored with matcha powder, which contains an amino acid called theanine that may help keep you mentally alert. Mango, kiwi, and papaya provide antioxidant phytochemicals and natural sweetness.

Serves 4 **Prep time** 25 minutes, plus chilling **Cook time** 10 minutes

INGREDIENTS

2½ cups coconut milk
½ (½ oz; 12g) package of powdered gelatin
2 tbsp light brown sugar
½ tsp **matcha powder**
1 tbsp sunflower oil

FOR THE FRUIT SALAD

1 passion fruit
½ ripe **mango**, peeled and finely diced
1 ripe **kiwi**, finely diced
½ ripe **papaya**, peeled and finely diced

SPECIAL EQUIPMENT

4 (5fl oz;150ml) ramekins

METHOD

1 Transfer 3 tablespoons of the coconut milk to a medium heatproof bowl. Scatter the gelatin over the surface of the milk and whisk it in well, then let rest for 5 minutes. Meanwhile, heat the remaining coconut milk in a small, heavy-bottomed saucepan over low heat until it is hot, but not boiling.

2 When the coconut milk is hot, remove it from the heat and pour it over the gelatin mixture, whisking well to ensure that all the gelatin granules have dissolved. Whisk in the sugar and matcha powder until completely combined.

3 Rub the insides of the ramekins with a piece of paper towel dipped in the sunflower oil. Divide the coconut mixture between the ramekins and allow the mixture to cool before transferring to the fridge for at least 4–6 hours, until set.

4 To make the fruit salad, cut the passion fruit in half and scrape the seeds out into a bowl. Mix the diced fruit with the passion fruit seeds and set aside.

5 To serve the panna cottas, fill a bowl with hot water and carefully dip the outside of each ramekin briefly into the water to loosen the panna cotta, being careful not to allow the water to drip onto the set cream. Run a small knife around the edge of the panna cotta and turn onto individual serving plates. Serve with the fruit salad.

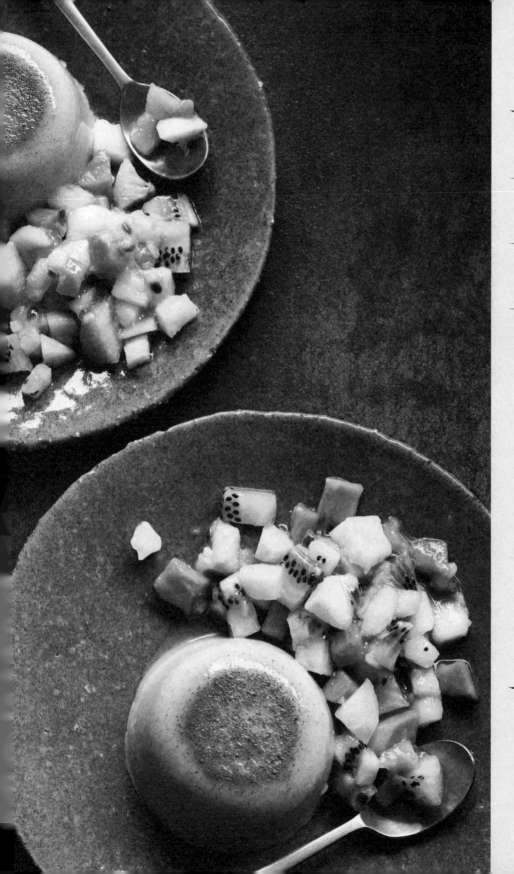

FEATURED SUPERFOODS

MATCHA POWDER
helps keep your
brain alert

MANGO
may help reduce the risk
of certain types of **cancer**

KIWI
helps keep your
skin healthy

PAPAYA
helps maintain
digestive health

Nutrition per serving

Energy 352cals (1427kj)
Carbohydrate 19g
– of which sugars 17g
Fiber 3g
Fat 28g
– of which saturated 22g
Salt 0g
Protein 4g
Cholesterol 0g

MANGO

High in vitamin C, which is essential for healthy bones and skin, mango is also rich in a group of phytochemicals that may help reduce the risk of certain types of cancer.

WHY EAT IT?

CANCER PREVENTION

Mangoes contain two groups of phytochemicals—carotenoids and polyphenols—that have been linked with a reduced risk of certain types of cancer, including prostate, colon, and breast cancers.

EYE HEALTH

The phytochemicals beta-carotene and zeaxanthin, which give mangoes their vibrant color, help protect the eyes from damage by free radicals. Mangoes are also a useful source of vitamin A, which is essential for healthy skin and eyes.

Ripe mangoes have a fruity fragrance at the end of the stems

WHAT'S IN IT?

1 medium mango (5½oz/150g) is a good source of vitamins C, A, and B6, as well as potassium. Mango also contains niacin, folate, and vitamin E.

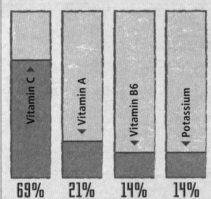

Vitamin C	Vitamin A	Vitamin B6	Potassium
69%	21%	14%	14%

Percentage of your daily reference intake

WHERE IS IT FROM?

Mangoes were first grown in India over 5,000 years ago and are now cultivated in many tropical and subtropical regions. They belong to the same family as coconuts, olives, and dates.

The skin color ranges from green to red or orange

HOW TO EAT IT

1 MANGO SALSA

Choose slightly firm mangoes to make salsa, rather than juicy ones, as they will hold their shape better when cutting. Add finely diced mango, scallions, mint, red bell pepper, and lime juice to a bowl and toss together before serving.

2 IN A SORBET

Sweeten blended mango with a little honey and a squeeze of lime juice. Churn in an ice-cream maker for a sensational superfood sorbet.

3 MANGO AND LIME TAPIOCA

Mango purée can be used to flavor many different types of simple dishes. Try blending it into a tapioca pudding with lime zest and juice.

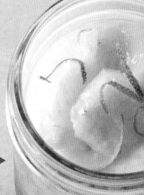

Mango and lime tapioca ▶

KIWI

Rich in vitamin C, which helps maintain healthy skin, kiwi is also high in certain phytochemicals that may protect the eyes from UV radiation.

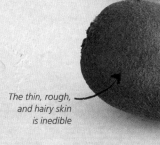

The thin, rough, and hairy skin is inedible

WHY EAT IT?

SKIN HEALTH
Kiwi contains vitamin C, which is essential for the manufacture of collagen, a protein that supports healthy skin. A study that assessed skin aging in over 4,025 women found that women with the highest intake of vitamin C had fewer wrinkles.

EYE HEALTH
Kiwi is rich in a phytochemical called lutein, an antioxidant that protects the eyes from UV radiation in sunlight and free radicals that can increase the risk of age-related macular degeneration (AMD).

MAXIMIZE THE BENEFITS

GOLDEN AND GREEN KIWI
Golden kiwi fruit contains more vitamin C than green, but green kiwi is richer in lutein and fiber. Vitamin C helps the body to absorb iron from foods like breakfast cereals. Add some kiwi slices to your cereal to help boost iron absorption.

WHAT'S IN IT?

1 kiwi (2oz/60g) is a good source of vitamins C and K, as well as folate and potassium.

Vitamin C	Vitamin K	Folate	Potassium
92%	32%	10%	9%

Percentage of your daily reference intake

WHERE IS IT FROM?

Native to China, kiwi fruits, or Chinese gooseberries, were first cultivated in New Zealand in the twentieth century and are now cultivated in other temperate regions.

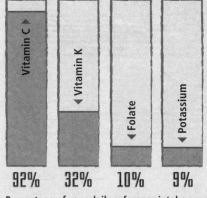

Sugar level in the fruit is measured to determine the harvest time

HOW TO EAT IT

1 FRUIT SALAD
Fruit salads can sometimes be too sweet—add kiwi fruits in a strawberry or banana salad for a sharp contrast in flavor. Kiwi also adds contrasting color, vitamins, and phytochemicals.

2 HOMEMADE ICE POPS
When the weather is hot, homemade ice pops are a healthy way to cool down. Blend peeled kiwis and freeze them in a ice pop mold. You could also add apple juice before freezing.

3 ADD TO SMOOTHIES
Kiwi fruit adds welcome sweetness to a traditional green smoothie, as well as plentiful quantities of vitamin C. Add 1 peeled kiwi to your usual mix of greens and blend until smooth.

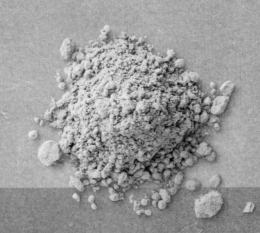

HERBS, SPICES, & POWDERS

TURMERIC

The star component of this vibrant yellow spice is curcumin, a potent phytochemical that has anti-inflammatory and antioxidant properties, and may help relieve arthritis symptoms, aid digestion, and inhibit the growth of cancers.

WHY EAT IT?

BONE STRENGTH
Curcumin, the active ingredient in turmeric, is known to have anti-inflammatory properties, and some studies suggest it can help relieve pain associated with tendonitis and arthritis.

BLOOD HEALTH
New research suggests that turmeric may help control blood pressure by relaxing the blood vessels, and reduce the risk of dementia by preventing the build-up of amyloid plaques, which restrict blood flow to the brain.

CANCER PREVENTION
Turmeric's antioxidant properties may have the potential to protect against certain cancers. One study found that curcumin may inhibit the size and number of precancerous polyps in the colon. Another study found that curcumin may help suppress cell proliferation in breast- and lung-cancer cells.

Turmeric contains **anti-inflammatory curcumin**, which can help **ease** the symptoms of **tendonitis** and **arthritis**.

WHAT'S IN IT?

A 1-tablespoon serving of ground turmeric provides a useful source of iron, manganese, potassium, and copper. Turmeric also contains phosphorus.

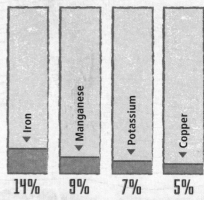

Iron	Manganese	Potassium	Copper
14%	9%	7%	5%

Percentage of your daily reference intake

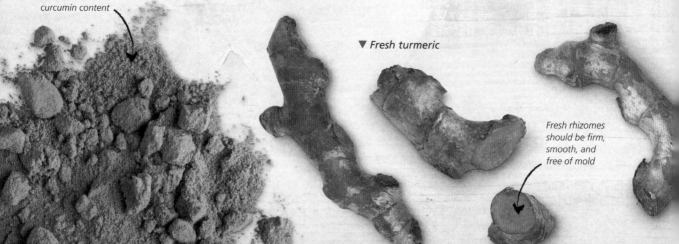

Turmeric's bright color comes from its curcumin content

▼ *Ground turmeric*

▼ *Fresh turmeric*

Fresh rhizomes should be firm, smooth, and free of mold

WHERE IS IT FROM?

Prized as a medicinal and culinary spice for at least 2,500 years in its native regions of South and Southeast Asia, turmeric is a member of the ginger family. The plant is cultivated for its aromatic rhizomes, which are stems that grow underground. Like ginger, turmeric rhizomes can be used fresh, but are often sold dried and ground for a longer shelf life. It is cultivated in tropical climates globally, with India being the world's largest producer.

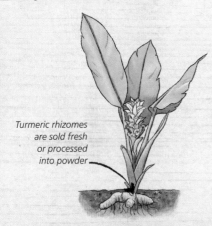

Turmeric rhizomes are sold fresh or processed into powder

MAXIMIZE THE BENEFITS

COOK OR SERVE WITH FAT
Curcumin is fat-soluble, so eating turmeric with a small amount of fat or oil helps your body to absorb it better.

EAT WITH ONIONS OR CAULIFLOWER
Early studies suggest that eating turmeric with quercetin-rich onions or with cruciferous vegetables, such as cauliflower, may help protect against colon and prostate cancers respectively.

HOW TO EAT IT

1 TURMERIC SCRAMBLE
A pinch of dried turmeric in a tofu or egg scramble gives it a wonderful golden color. Include bright vegetables, such as sautéed red and green bell peppers, for extra nutrient value.

2 IN JUICE
Add peeled and finely grated fresh turmeric to a carrot, orange, and ginger smoothie for a colorful, refreshing drink.

3 TURMERIC LATTE
Steep fresh turmeric in boiling water or hot milk to help extract its colorful curcumin. Alternatively, use 1 teaspoon of ground turmeric and strain before drinking. Add honey to taste.

The **antioxidant** properties of **turmeric** may help **prevent** the formation of **cancerous cells** in the **colon**, **breasts**, and **lungs**.

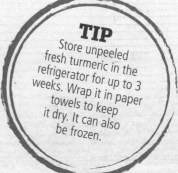

TIP
Store unpeeled fresh turmeric in the refrigerator for up to 3 weeks. Wrap it in paper towels to keep it dry. It can also be frozen.

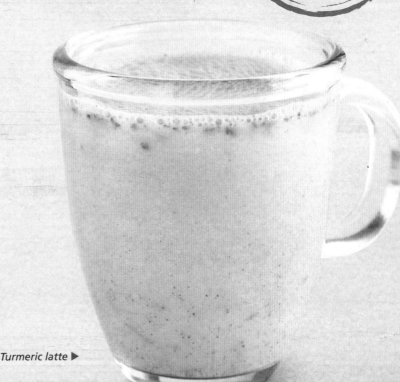

Turmeric latte ▶

SWEET POTATO & SPINACH CURRY

Based on sweet potatoes, baby spinach, and coconut milk, this vitamin C–rich dish is then flavored with superfood spices. Mustard seeds and turmeric have anti-inflammatory properties, while cinnamon helps control blood sugar.

Serves 4   **Prep time** 10 minutes   **Cook time** 20 minutes

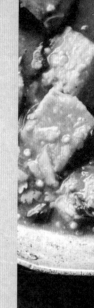

INGREDIENTS

2 tbsp coconut oil

1 **onion**, finely chopped

2 cloves **garlic**, crushed

1 piece of **ginger**, about
   2in (5cm), grated

1 tsp **mustard seeds**

1/4 tsp ground **cinnamon**

1/2 tsp **turmeric** powder

1/2 tsp **cayenne pepper**

1 tsp ground **cumin**

1 tsp ground **coriander**

1 (14oz; 400ml) can
   reduced-fat coconut milk

1 cup low-sodium
   vegetable stock

3 large **sweet potatoes**,
   peeled and cut into
   1 1/2in (3cm) cubes, about
   1 1/2lb (700g) in total

3 cups baby **spinach** leaves

1 small handful **cilantro** leaves,
   coarsely chopped

METHOD

1 Heat the coconut oil in a large, shallow pan. Cook the onion over medium heat for 3–4 minutes, until it has softened but is not brown. Add the garlic and ginger and cook for another minute, then add all the remaining spices and cook over low heat for another minute, stirring constantly, until they darken slightly and start to release their fragrance.

2 Add the coconut milk and vegetable stock to the pan and mix well. Add the diced sweet potatoes and bring the mixture to a boil, then reduce to a low simmer and cook, covered, for 10–12 minutes until the potatoes are just soft.

3 Remove the lid and gently stir in the spinach leaves to avoid breaking up the sweet potatoes. The curry is ready when the spinach has wilted into the sauce, which should take about 1–2 minutes. Taste and add a little salt, if needed.

4 Remove from the heat and stir in the chopped cilantro before serving with cooked brown rice.

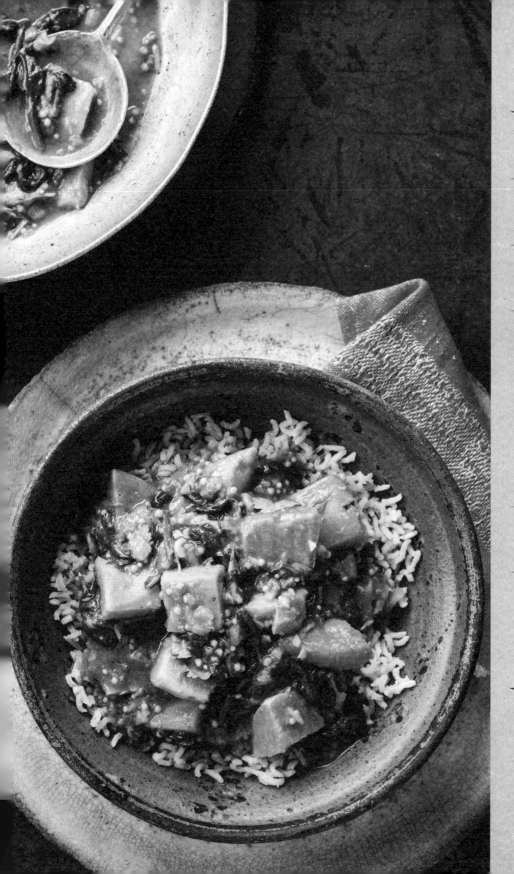

FEATURED SUPERFOODS

ONIONS
encourage the growth
of **gut-friendly bacteria**

GARLIC
may deactivate
cancer-causing agents

GINGER
lowers the risk of
high blood pressure

SPICES
- **Mustard seeds**
  are antioxidant
- **Cinnamon** helps
  control blood sugar
- **Turmeric** is
  anti-inflammatory
- **Cayenne pepper** may
  boost your metabolism
- **Cumin** aids digestion
- **Coriander** helps keep
  your skin and eyes healthy

SWEET POTATOES
help maintain your
immune system

SPINACH
may help protect
your **eyes**

Nutrition per serving

Energy 336cals (1336kj)

Carbohydrate 40g
– of which sugars 13g

Fiber 7g

Fat 16g
– of which saturated 13g

Salt 0.3g

Protein 4.5g

Cholesterol 0g

CAYENNE PEPPER

This pungent spice owes its superfood status to capsaicin, an antibacterial phytochemical that supports digestive health. Cayenne may also help improve circulation.

WHY EAT IT?

DISEASE PREVENTION
Capsaicin, the phytochemical that gives cayenne its spicy taste, has antiviral, antibacterial, and antidiabetic properties, and may help relieve pain.

DIGESTIVE HEALTH
The capsaicin in cayenne pepper may help prevent stomach ulcers by helping your body produce mucus that protects the stomach lining. Some research suggests that capsaicin boosts your metabolism, helping burn excess fats.

HEART HEALTH
Research suggests that cayenne may improve circulation and lower high blood pressure. This helps keep your arteries clear of blood clots, reducing the risk of heart disease and stroke.

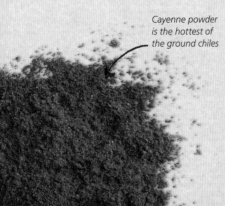

Cayenne powder is the hottest of the ground chiles

WHAT'S IN IT?

2 tablespoons of cayenne pepper is a good source of vitamin A, as well as manganese, potassium, and vitamin B2. Cayenne also contains vitamin B1, niacin, and magnesium.

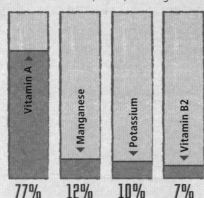

Vitamin A	Manganese	Potassium	Vitamin B2
77%	12%	10%	7%

Percentage of your daily reference intake

WHERE IS IT FROM?

Cayenne pepper is the fruit of a plant in the nightshade family. It is native to tropical regions of the Americas.

The green fruit turns bright red when ripe

HOW TO EAT IT

1 HOT DRINK
Start your day with a refreshing drink of hot water seasoned with honey, lemon, and a pinch of cayenne pepper.

2 IN A MARINADE
Whisk cayenne pepper with olive oil, lemon juice, salt, and pepper, and use as a quick, sweet-and-spicy basting sauce for grilled meat or fish.

3 ROMESCO SAUCE
Combine roasted red bell peppers with 1–2 teaspoons of cayenne pepper, a handful of blanched almonds, and a little garlic and olive oil. Blend to a thick paste and use as a dip or in a sandwich or wrap.

TIP
Dry your own cayenne peppers by slicing them lengthwise and heating them in a low oven for 6–8 hours. Use whole or process to a powder.

CINNAMON

Rich in energy-boosting manganese, cinnamon is also antibacterial and may protect your brain against Alzheimer's disease.

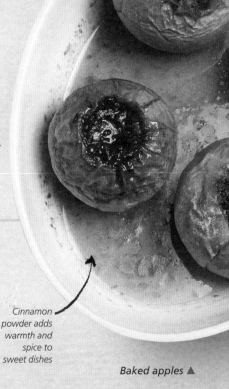

WHY EAT IT?

ENERGY BALANCE
Recent research suggests that cinnamon can slow the absorption of sugar, helping to avoid spikes in blood sugar.

DISEASE PREVENTION
Cinnamaldehyde, an active ingredient in cinnamon, is believed to have antibacterial and antifungal properties. Antioxidants in cinnamon may also reduce inflammation.

BRAIN POWER
Research from Tel Aviv University suggests that compounds found in cinnamon may lower the risk of Alzheimer's disease. It is thought to work by inhibiting the production of a type of protein associated with the disease.

WHAT'S IN IT?

3 tablespoons of cinnamon powder is a great source of manganese, as well as iron, copper, and potassium. Cinnamon also contains zinc, magnesium, and calcium, as well as vitamins B6 and K.

Manganese ▲	Iron ▼	Copper ▼	Potassium ▼
218%	15%	9%	5%

Percentage of your daily reference intake

Cinnamon powder adds warmth and spice to sweet dishes

Baked apples ▲

HOW TO EAT IT

1 BAKED APPLES
For a simple dessert, stuff cored apples with a mixture of dried fruit, nuts, and ground cinnamon, and bake in a medium oven until softened and fragrant.

2 IN BREAKFAST
Cinnamon powder makes a flavorful addition to breakfast foods. Try mixing it into oatmeal, adding to a smoothie, or using as a flavoring for homemade granola (see pp24–25).

3 CINNAMON BANANA CHIPS
Make your own banana chips by tossing thin slices of firm banana in lemon juice and ground cinnamon and baking in a low oven until completely dried out. Eat as a snack or use as a topping for oatmeal.

WHERE IS IT FROM?

Cinnamon is a small tree that is native to southeast Asia. The bark is dried for culinary use.

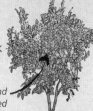

The branches and trunks are harvested for their flavorful bark

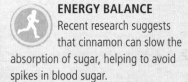

Quills of cinnamon bark are used whole or ground into powder

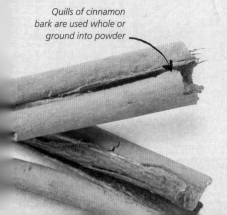

GINGER

Ginger contains at least 14 phytochemicals, many of which have impressive antioxidant and anti-inflammatory properties. It is also a good source of copper, which supports your bones, blood, and nervous system.

WHY EAT IT?

NAUSEA PREVENTION
Several studies have shown that ginger—in fresh or powdered form—can help to relieve nausea, including that associated with travel sickness, pregnancy, or chemotherapy treatments.

DIGESTIVE HEALTH
Naturopaths recommend eating ginger to treat a range of digestive problems, such as indigestion, flatulence, and bloating. Experts believe it works by boosting digestive juices and neutralizing acids.

HEART HEALTH
One study has revealed that regular consumption of ginger may lower the risk of developing high blood pressure, and reduce the risk of heart disease by 13 percent.

Good source of **COPPER**

Regular consumption of ginger may **lower** the risk of developing **high blood pressure** and also **reduce** the risk of **heart disease** by **13 percent.**

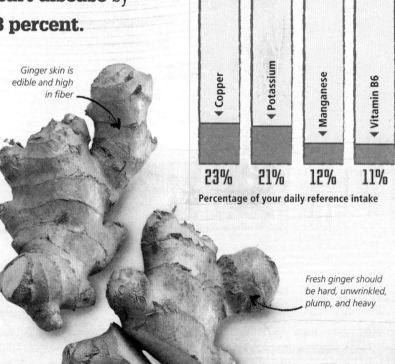

Ginger skin is edible and high in fiber

Fresh ginger should be hard, unwrinkled, plump, and heavy

WHAT'S IN IT?

1 cup of sliced ginger provides a useful source of copper, potassium, manganese, and vitamin B6. Ginger also contains vitamins C, B1, B2, and B3, as well as folate, magnesium, iron, and zinc.

▼ Copper	▼ Potassium	▼ Manganese	▼ Vitamin B6
23%	21%	12%	11%

Percentage of your daily reference intake

Both **fresh** and **powdered ginger** can help **relieve nausea**, including that associated with the early stages of **pregnancy**.

WHERE IS IT FROM?

Ginger is a member of *Zingiberaceae*—a botanical family that also includes turmeric and cardamom. Native to Southeast Asia, India, and China, it is the rhizome (underground stem) of a creeping perennial plant. It is now cultivated in many tropical countries and is available in myriad forms, including fresh, crystallized, pickled, and powdered.

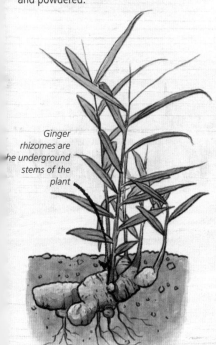

Ginger rhizomes are the underground stems of the plant

HOW TO EAT IT

1 GINGER AND MAPLE SHRUB
A shrub makes a great base for a nonalcoholic cocktail. Make a purée of apple cider vinegar, peeled fresh ginger, water, and a little maple syrup, then strain and dilute with sparkling water.

2 CURRY BASE
Gently crush cumin, coriander seeds, and cardamom pods in a mortar and pestle with freshly grated ginger. Cook the mixture with chopped onions in a little canola oil until softened and fragrant. Use as a base for meat or vegetable curries.

HOW TO PREPARE

The richest resins in ginger are just beneath the skin, so it's important to peel it with care. An easy way to do this is to scrape the skin with the tip of a teaspoon. You can also use a paring knife or vegetable peeler, but these remove more of the nutrient-rich flesh. Once peeled, finely slice, chop, or grate the ginger.

Gently scrape off the skin to preserve the nutrients in the flesh beneath

TIP
Store unpeeled fresh ginger in the fridge for up to 3 weeks, or freeze peeled and grated ginger to preserve freshness.

3 PAPAYA AND GINGER SMOOTHIE
Adding a teaspoon or two of grated fresh ginger to smoothies adds a warm, spicy kick. Ginger pairs especially well with carrot or papaya juice.

Papaya and ginger smoothie ▶

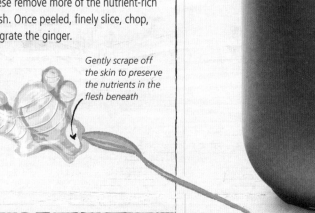

CUMIN

A rich source of blood-building iron, cumin may also help balance your blood sugar levels and reduce bad cholesterol. It is also traditionally used as a digestive aid.

WHY EAT IT?

DIGESTIVE HEALTH
Research suggests that cumin may aid digestion by stimulating the production of bile, which helps your body to digest fat.

BLOOD HEALTH
Early research from Mysore University in India suggests that cumin may have an antidiabetic effect by helping to lower blood sugar levels.

HEART HEALTH
Cumin is rich in phytochemicals including phytosterols, which are known to help lower levels of bad LDL cholesterol in your body.

Buy whole seeds and use them as they are or grind them to a powder

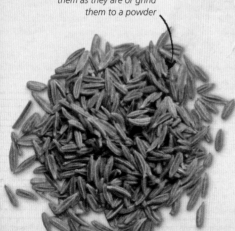

WHAT'S IN IT?

¼ cup of cumin seeds provides high quantities of iron and manganese, as well as potassium and vitamin B6. Cumin also contains vitamins B1, B2, and E, as well as copper, zinc, and magnesium.

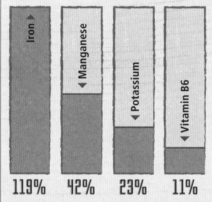

Iron ▲ | Manganese ▼ | Potassium ▼ | Vitamin B6 ▼

| 119% | 42% | 23% | 11% |

Percentage of your daily reference intake

WHERE IS IT FROM?

Native to the eastern Mediterranean region, cumin is the seed of a small plant in the parsley family.

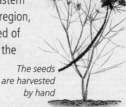

The seeds are harvested by hand

HOW TO EAT IT

1 CUMIN TEA
Make a soothing digestive tea by simmering a spoonful of cumin seeds in water for 5 minutes. Strain the liquid and sweeten with a little honey to serve.

2 IN A SPICE MIX
Create your own Indian-inspired spice mix using ground cumin, coriander, and turmeric. Dust it on whole fish before grilling, and serve with a squeeze of lime.

3 SPICED DIP
Blend the soft flesh of a baked sweet potato with a little cumin and honey to make a healthy dip for homemade flatbread chips.

TIP
Ground cumin loses its flavor quite quickly, so buy whole seeds and grind to a powder with a mortar and pestle just before use.

MUSTARD SEEDS

Packed with phytochemicals, mustard seeds may help reduce the risk of cancer and lower levels of bad cholesterol. They also contain bone-strengthening phosphorus.

WHY EAT IT?

CANCER PREVENTION
Glucosinolates, a group of phytochemicals present in mustard seeds, have been shown to inhibit the growth of cancer cells. Mustard seeds are also a useful source of selenium, which is known to lower the risk of certain cancers.

HEART HEALTH
Mustard seeds contain phytosterols, phytochemicals that compete with cholesterol for absorption in the gut, which helps to lower levels of bad cholesterol.

BONE STRENGTH
The seeds are a useful source of phosphorus, which combines with calcium to give your bones and teeth strength and rigidity.

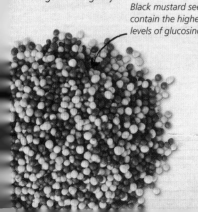

Black mustard seeds contain the highest levels of glucosinolates

WHAT'S IN IT?

¼ cup of mustard seeds provides high quantities of phosphorus, manganese, magnesium, and vitamin B1. Mustard seeds also contain vitamin B2, niacin, iron, zinc, potassium, selenium, and copper.

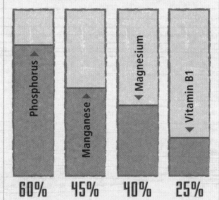

Phosphorus	Manganese	Magnesium	Vitamin B1
60%	45%	40%	25%

Percentage of your daily reference intake

WHERE IS IT FROM?

Cultivated since 3000 BCE, mustard seeds come from the pods of a flowering herb. Seeds are black, brown, yellow, or white in color.

Seedpods contain up to 20 seeds each

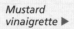

Mustard vinaigrette ▶

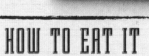

Toasted mustard seeds add a sharp burst of flavor

HOW TO EAT IT

1 MUSTARD VINAIGRETTE
Whisk toasted mustard seeds with ¾ cup of olive oil, 5 tbsp of white wine vinegar, 1 tsp of Dijon mustard, salt, and pepper to make a tangy vinaigrette.

2 HOMEMADE MUSTARD
Soak ½ cup of mustard seeds in ⅔ cup of vinegar and ½ cup of cold water for 2–3 days, until soft. Blend with a little honey until smooth.

3 SPROUT THEM
Add peppery mustard sprouts to salads. Soak the seeds first, then drain and rinse frequently until sprouts appear.

PARSLEY

An excellent source of vitamin K, as well as vitamin C, folate, and iron, parsley helps keep your bones and blood healthy, and protects your skin from damage by free radicals.

WHY EAT IT?

SKIN HEALTH
Weight for weight, fresh parsley contains three times more vitamin C than oranges. Vitamin C provides antioxidant protection from free radicals that can damage your skin.

BONE STRENGTH
Parsley is extraordinarily high in vitamin K, which helps the body to incorporate more calcium into the bones.

BLOOD HEALTH
Parsley contains a useful amount of iron and the B vitamin folate, both of which are needed for the manufacture of red blood cells.

WHAT'S IN IT?

1 tablespoon of fresh parsley provides an excellent source of vitamins K and C, folate, and iron. Parsley also contains vitamins A and B1, as well as potassium.

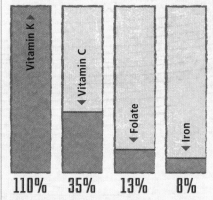

Vitamin K	Vitamin C	Folate	Iron
110%	35%	13%	8%

Percentage of your daily reference intake

HOW TO EAT IT

1 **ADD TO SOUP**
Add a large handful of chopped young parsley to a spring vegetable soup for added color, flavor, and nutrients.

2 **MIX IN A SMOOTHIE**
Blend a handful of flat-leaf parsley with kale, spinach, and celery for a glassful of green goodness.

3 **SALSA VERDE**
The Italians pair *salsa verde* (green salsa) with grilled meats and fish. To make it, blend parsley, mint, and basil with garlic and olive oil, and season to taste.

WHERE IS IT FROM?

A versatile herb, parsley is native to the eastern Mediterranean region. Today it is cultivated throughout most of the temperate world. Parsley is an easy-to-grow biennial plant in mild climates, and an annual in cold climates. There are two types—flat-leaf and curly. Many prefer the fine flavor of the flat-leaf variety, especially when it is cooked.

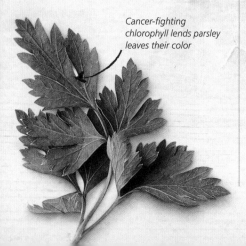

Cancer-fighting chlorophyll lends parsley leaves their color

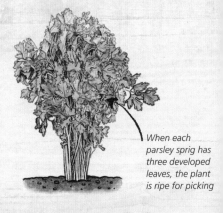

When each parsley sprig has three developed leaves, the plant is ripe for picking

MINT

Fresh mint is antioxidant and anti-inflammatory, and can have a calming effect on the digestive system. It is also a good source of folate, which supports blood health.

WHY EAT IT?

DIGESTIVE HEALTH
Menthol and methyl salicylate—two of the active ingredients in peppermint—have antispasmodic and calming effects on the muscles of the digestive tract. Peppermint can help relieve trapped gas in the stomach and improve the flow of bile—helping the body to digest fats.

IMMUNE BOOST
Mint contains antioxidant and anti-inflammatory rosmarinic acid, which may help relieve the symptoms of hay fever. It also contains menthol—a natural decongestant that can provide relief from the symptoms of coughs and colds.

Fresh mint leaves contain more nutrients than dried leaves

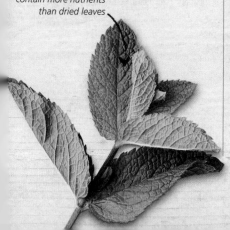

WHAT'S IN IT?

3½oz (100g) of fresh mint provides a good source of folate, calcium, vitamin B2, and potassium.

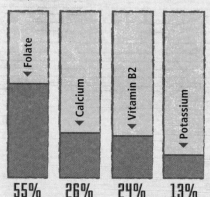

Folate	Calcium	Vitamin B2	Potassium
55%	26%	24%	13%

Percentage of your daily reference intake

WHERE IS IT FROM?

Native to southern Europe and the Mediterranean, mint has long grown wild all over the temperate world.

Growers harvest mint shortly before it flowers, when essential oils are strong

Freezing fresh mint leaves preserves their nutrients

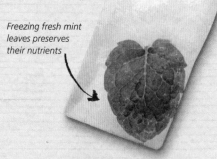

▲ *Mint ice cubes*

HOW TO EAT IT

1 MINT ICE CUBES
Add fresh mint leaves, whole or chopped, to an ice cube tray, fill with filtered water, and freeze. Add the frozen cubes to water or fruit juice for a hint of mint flavor, or defrost in a strainer or cheesecloth and use as you would fresh mint.

2 MINT INFUSION
A cup of mint tea can help with digestion after a meal. Steep the fresh leaves in boiling water for 5 minutes and sweeten with a little honey if needed.

3 ASIAN-STYLE SALAD
Fresh herbs make a welcome addition to all kinds of Asian-inspired salads. Dress shredded vegetables with finely chopped chile, lime juice, and a little olive oil, and mix with plenty of fresh mint.

HERBED TABBOULEH

A celebration of superfood herbs, this Middle Eastern–style salad is packed with fresh parsley and mint. These herbs are rich in vitamins K and C, and manganese, supporting your skeletal, circulatory, nervous, and immune systems.

Serves 4   Prep time 30 minutes, plus soaking

INGREDIENTS

1 cup bulgur wheat

½ red **onion**, peeled and very finely diced

salt and freshly ground black pepper

¾ cup flat-leaf **parsley**, leaves only, finely chopped

¾ cup **mint** leaves, finely chopped

¼ cup **lemon** juice

¼ cup extra-virgin olive oil

2 ripe **tomatoes**, seeded and finely diced

METHOD

1 Rinse the bulgur wheat through a strainer under running water, then put it in a large bowl. Cover with plenty of cold water and let soak for at least 2 hours, until it is soft. Drain well and set aside.

2 Place the diced onion in a salad bowl and season well with salt and pepper. Massage it with your fingers for a minute to soften the onion—the salt will draw out some of the vegetable's juices.

3 Add the chopped herbs to the onion, along with the lemon juice and olive oil, and toss together well. Add the bulgur wheat and chopped tomatoes and mix once more to combine all the ingredients well.

4 The salad can be served immediately but, if possible, cover and chill for up to 4 hours to allow the flavors to develop. Toss and check the seasoning before serving.

SUPER SWAP

Replace the bulgur wheat with steamed and drained cauliflower rice (see p112) for a tasty gluten-free and carb-free alternative.

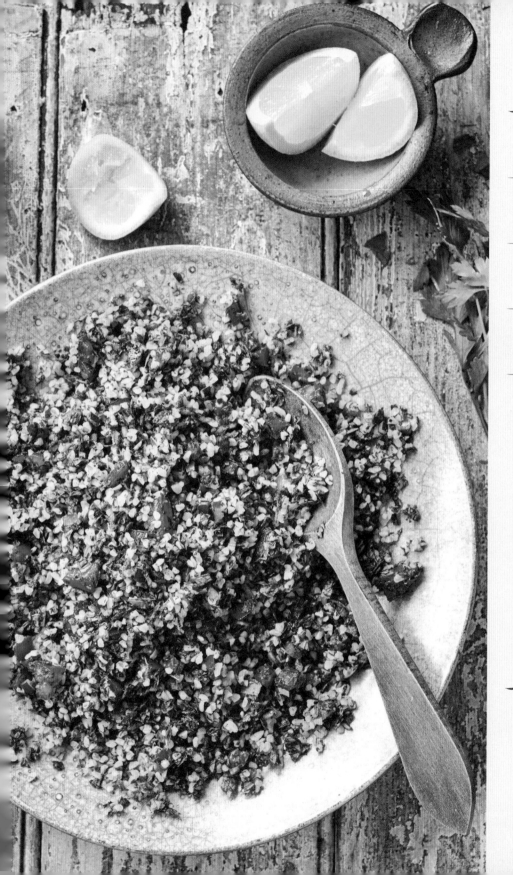

FEATURED SUPERFOODS

ONIONS
encourage the growth
of **gut-friendly bacteria**

PARSLEY
helps maintain
healthy bones

MINT
helps boost your
immune system

LEMON
helps maintain your
immune system

TOMATOES
may reduce the risk of
heart-related diseases

Nutrition
per serving

Energy 243cals (975kj)
Carbohydrate 27g
– of which sugars 4g
Fiber 4g
Fat 12g
– of which saturated 2g
Salt 0g
Protein 5g
Cholesterol 0g

ROSEMARY

Rosemary provides blood-healthy iron, as well as phytochemicals that may help protect against cognitive decline, slow the growth of cancer, and protect your eyes.

WHY EAT IT?

BRAIN POWER
Rosemary contains cineole, a phytochemical that is thought to prevent the breakdown of acetylcholine in the brain. Acetylcholine enables nerve cells to communicate with each other, and its decline with age is thought to cause loss of memory and mental agility. Carnosic acid, another phytochemical in rosemary, is believed to neutralize free radicals before they can cause damage in the brain.

DISEASE PREVENTION
Studies suggest that the various phytochemicals in rosemary may inhibit the growth of cancer cells. One such phytochemical, carnosic acid, also protects the eyes from free-radical damage.

BLOOD HEALTH
Rosemary is a useful source of iron, which your body needs to build the red blood cells that carry oxygen. Iron deficiency is a common cause of lethargy.

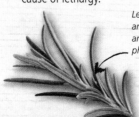

Leaves contain antioxidant and anti-inflammatory phytochemicals

WHAT'S IN IT?

3½oz (100g) of fresh rosemary provides good quantities of iron, calcium, vitamin B6, and manganese. Rosemary also contains zinc, potassium, and folate.

Iron	Calcium	Vitamin B6	Manganese
61%	36%	31%	27%

Percentage of your daily reference intake

WHERE IS IT FROM?

Rosemary is a shrub in the mint family, originating from the Mediterranean region. Its leaves are used fresh or dried.

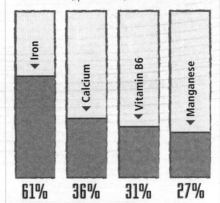

The needlelike leaves are evergreen

HOW TO EAT IT

1 WITH POTATOES
Rosemary and potatoes are a match made in heaven. Simply toss sliced new potatoes in garlic, rosemary, and olive oil, and roast them until crisp.

2 ROSEMARY-BAKED FRUIT
Add complexity to a simple dish of baked apricots or plums. Place a sprig of rosemary in the baking dish, top with the pitted fruit, and roast until soft and fragrant.

3 INFUSED OIL
Add a couple of fresh rosemary stalks to a bottle of olive oil and wait a week to infuse. Use the infused oil to flavor all types of meat, fish, and vegetable dishes.

Discard the woody stalk, as it is inedible

THYME

Rich in energy-boosting manganese and anti-inflammatory phytochemicals, thyme may help keep your blood and immune system healthy.

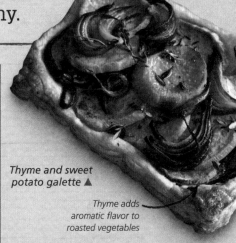

Thyme and sweet potato galette ▲

Thyme adds aromatic flavor to roasted vegetables

WHY EAT IT?

DISEASE PREVENTION

Thyme contains a number of phytochemicals, including thymol and carvacrol, which have been shown to have anti-inflammatory properties. Thyme is thought to help strengthen your immune system and protect against cancer.

BLOOD HEALTH

Early studies suggest that thyme may have strong antioxidative properties that help to reduce blood pressure and lower cholesterol.

DIGESTIVE HEALTH

Thyme is believed to help aid digestion by stimulating the liver to produce digestive enzymes.

WHAT'S IN IT?

3½oz (100g) of fresh thyme provides high quantities of manganese, calcium, folate, and zinc, as well as vitamins B1, B6, and C, magnesium, phosphorus, and niacin.

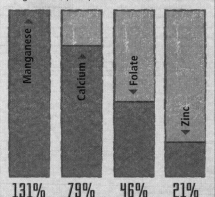

Manganese ▲	Calcium ▶	◀ Folate	◀ Zinc
131%	79%	46%	21%

Percentage of your daily reference intake

WHERE IS IT FROM?

Native to Eurasia, thyme is related to mint. The leaves are harvested and sold fresh or dried.

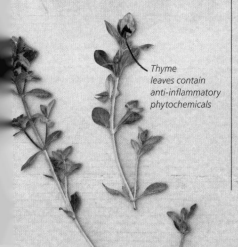

Small leaves grow on woody stems

Thyme leaves contain anti-inflammatory phytochemicals

HOW TO EAT IT

1 THYME AND SWEET POTATO GALETTE
To make a tasty galette laden with superfoods, sprinkle thyme over cooked sweet potatoes and red onion on a puff pastry base, and bake until golden.

2 HOT DRINK
For a soothing, aromatic drink, steep sprigs of fresh or dried thyme in hot water, and add honey and lemon juice to taste.

3 ADD TO VEGETABLES
Thyme is a strongly flavored, woody herb and is best used sparingly and always cooked, unless the leaves are very young. Scatter thyme over a variety of chopped root vegetables before roasting.

CILANTRO

A good source of bone-strengthening vitamin K, cilantro (known as coriander when ground) is also rich in antioxidants that help protect the eyes from damage by free radicals.

WHY EAT IT?

DIGESTIVE HEALTH
Cilantro has traditionally been used to soothe a troubled digestive system. Studies show it can inhibit the formation of heterocyclic amines (HCA), carcinogenic compounds that are created when meat is cooked at very high temperatures.

EYE HEALTH
Cilantro contains carotenoids, including beta-carotene, lutein, and zeaxanthin, antioxidants that protect the eyes from free radicals and reduce the risk of cataracts and age-related macular degeneration (AMD).

HIGH IN VITAMIN K
Vitamin K is important for strong bones and healthy blood. Low levels of vitamin K have been associated with increased risk of osteoporosis.

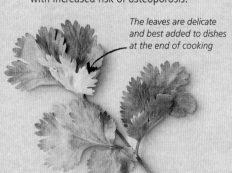

The leaves are delicate and best added to dishes at the end of cooking

WHAT'S IN IT?

A small bunch of fresh cilantro provides an excellent source of vitamin K and a good source of vitamin C, folate, and potassium.

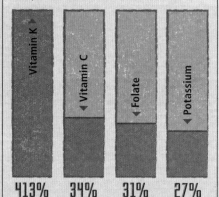

Vitamin K — 413%
Vitamin C — 34%
Folate — 31%
Potassium — 27%

Percentage of your daily reference intake

WHERE IS IT FROM?

Native to Mediterranean and Western Asia, cilantro is grown worldwide. It is an annual herb belonging to the *Apiaceae* family that is used as a herb and spice.

All parts of the plant, from roots to leaves, are edible

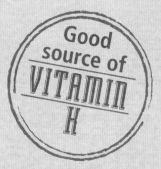

HOW TO EAT IT

1 HERB SALAD
A fresh herb salad makes the best accompaniment to all kinds of grilled meats and fish. Mix handfuls of fresh Italian parsley, cilantro, and mint leaves and dress with a citrusy vinaigrette.

2 IN SOUP
Carrot and cilantro soup is a classic flavour combination for soup. Make an extra-flavorful version by using both ground coriander—as a spice in the soup—and chopped fresh cilantro, for garnish.

3 ADD TO CURRY PASTE
The stalks and roots of fresh cilantro are often overlooked, yet they are invaluable when making your own Asian-inspired spice pastes. Use chopped cilantro stems in a Thai green curry paste.

Good source of **VITAMIN K**

MATCHA POWDER

Matcha powder is rich in a group of antioxidants called polyphenols, which are believed to lower the risk of heart disease and certain types of cancer.

WHY EAT IT?

CANCER PREVENTION
A number of studies suggest that drinking matcha tea may reduce the risk of certain types of cancer, including colon, breast, ovary, prostate, and lung cancers. It contains catechins, a group of phytochemicals that are believed to slow or halt the growth of cancer cells.

ENERGY BALANCE
Matcha contains epigallocatechin gallate (EGCG), a phytochemical that may help speed up your metabolism. Some research suggests that matcha tea may be helpful if you are trying to lose weight, as it may help boost your metabolism during exercise.

BRAIN POWER
Matcha powder contains high levels of the amino acid theanine, which may improve brain function. Theanine is believed to work by reducing the effects of stress while simultaneously keeping your brain alert. Matcha also contains caffeine, which helps your mind stay alert and focused.

WHAT'S IN IT?

1 scant teaspoon of matcha powder provides good quantities of vitamins K, A, B2, and B1. Matcha also contains magnesium and potassium.

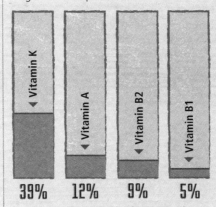

Vitamin K	Vitamin A	Vitamin B2	Vitamin B1
39%	**12%**	**9%**	**5%**

Percentage of your daily reference intake

WHERE IS IT FROM?

Made from the leaf tips of the tea plant, *Camellia sinensis*, matcha is a shrub native to southern China.

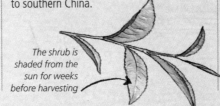

The shrub is shaded from the sun for weeks before harvesting

HOW TO EAT IT

1 **BREAKFAST BOWL**
Enhance your morning yogurt with a little matcha powder stirred in or simply sprinkled on top, along with some chopped fruit and a handful of granola.

2 **FOR ADDED FLAVOR**
Use a little matcha powder to flavor all kinds of milk-based desserts, smoothies, and milkshakes. Matcha powder also gives them a delicate greenish hue.

3 **MATCHA TEA**
Matcha powder is derived from green tea leaves, and can be used to make an instant version of green tea. Simply dilute it with boiling water, and sweeten to taste with some honey.

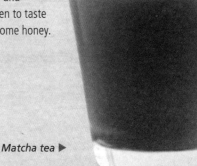

Matcha tea ▶

MORINGA POWDER

A super source of bone-strenghening vitamin K and energy-boosting iron, moringa powder also contains more than 50 antioxidants and phytochemicals that help fight disease.

WHY EAT IT?

ENERGY BALANCE
Moringa's high iron content may explain its traditional use as an herbal remedy for fatigue, which is a common symptom of iron deficiency.

DISEASE PREVENTION
The numerous phytochemicals in moringa include quercetin and chlorogenic acid. One study found that taking the powder regularly can boost the body's levels of antioxidants, which help neutralize the free radicals that cause cell damage and can lead to cancerous growths.

BLOOD HEALTH
Early research suggests that moringa may have anti-diabetic properties that help reduce blood sugar levels after a meal.

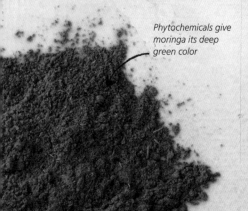
Phytochemicals give moringa its deep green color

WHAT'S IN IT?

2 tablespoons of moringa powder is an excellent source of vitamin K and iron, as well as vitamin A and calcium. It also contains magnesium, phosphorus, and zinc.

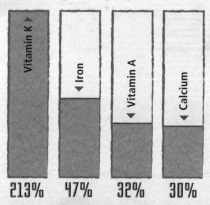

Vitamin K	Iron	Vitamin A	Calcium
213%	47%	32%	30%

Percentage of your daily reference intake

WHERE IS IT FROM?

Native to the Himalayas, moringa is a deciduous tree that grows in tropical regions of Asia and the Americas. It is also known as the horseradish tree because of its strongly flavored roots. The trees grow to about 30ft (9m) in height and produce bright green, fern-shaped leaves, from which the powder is made.

HOW TO EAT IT

1 IN TEA
Moringa powder has a beautiful green color, and is traditionally made into a tea. Dissolve 1 teaspoon of powder in boiling water and sweeten with honey to taste.

2 GREEN SMOOTHIE
Add 1 teaspoon of moringa powder to kale- or spinach-based smoothies for a colorful, iron-rich drink.

3 ICE POPS
Add 2 teaspoons of moringa powder to juiced apples, oranges, and cucumber, mix well, and freeze in molds to create nutritious citrus ice pops.

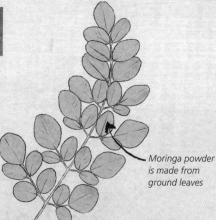
Moringa powder is made from ground leaves

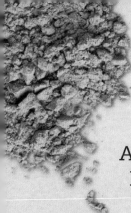

MACA POWDER

A good source of iodine, maca powder aids hormone balance and helps regulate your metabolism. Maca also contains blood-healthy iron and B vitamins.

WHY EAT IT?

ENERGY BALANCE
Maca is believed to boost energy levels. It contains iron, the raw material for oxygen-carrying hemoglobin; vitamin B6, which helps your body make red blood cells; and vitamin B2, which releases energy from food.

HORMONE BALANCE
Iodine helps in the manufacture of thyroid hormones, which are needed for many bodily processes such as growth and regulating metabolism. Traditionally, maca was thought by the Incas to enhance fertility, and early research suggests that maca may increase sperm production in some men.

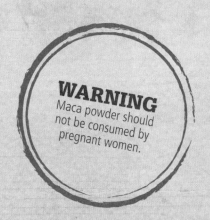

WARNING
Maca powder should not be consumed by pregnant women.

WHAT'S IN IT?

2 tablespoons of maca powder is a source of iodine, iron, potassium, and vitamin B6, as well as copper, manganese, vitamin B2, magnesium, selenium, niacin, and calcium.

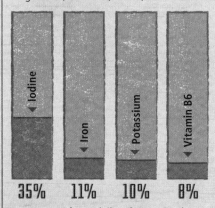

Iodine	Iron	Potassium	Vitamin B6
35%	11%	10%	8%

Percentage of your daily reference intake

WHERE IS IT FROM?

Grown as a versatile vegetable in the Peruvian Andes for more than 3,000 years, maca root is commonly exported as powder.

The root is dried and ground to make powder

HOW TO EAT IT

1 IN ENERGY BARS
Maca powder has a rich, malty taste that gives a boost to raw energy bars. Blend dried fruit, nuts, seeds, and 1 tablespoon of maca powder into a stiff mixture and spread it in a baking sheet. Allow it to firm up in the refrigerator, then cut into bars.

2 ADD TO BROWNIES
Enhance a brownie recipe (see p58) with a spoonful of this power powder. Cacao and maca are a delicious pairing.

3 MACA SMOOTHIE
Whip up a tasty banana smoothie with Greek yogurt, apple, a pinch of cinnamon, and 1 teaspoon of maca powder for a gently warming, malty flavor.

Maca smoothie ▶

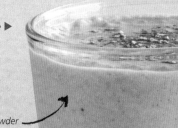

Maca powder adds malty flavor to smoothies

EATING FOR ENERGY

Adding superfoods into your diet can aid you in your quest to stay vibrant and alert, as they are packed with energy-boosting nutrients and healthy, slow-release energy. Here is an example of a day of eating to boost and balance your energy levels.

MID-MORNING SNACK

Around 3 hours after breakfast, your blood sugar levels may start to drop, causing a dip in energy levels. To prevent this from happening, eat a small, nutritious snack: a handful of fresh or dried fruit, or whole-grain crackers spread with nut butter are good choices.

TO DRINK

Your body can become slightly dehydrated overnight, leaving you feeling sluggish in the morning. Drink a large glass of water or a small glass of fruit juice to jump-start your morning.

Fruit juice is rehydrating and rich in vitamins

BREAKFAST

Never skip breakfast, as this meal will provide you with the energy you need for the morning. Oatmeal or muesli are excellent choices: the carbohydrates in oats break down slowly, staving off hunger pangs for the entire morning. You can also add a handful of oats to a smoothie for an easy breakfast.

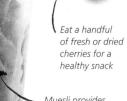

Eat a handful of fresh or dried cherries for a healthy snack

Muesli provides energy-balancing, slow-release carbohydrates

Stay hydrated
Lethargy and fatigue are a common sign that your body is dehydrated, so drink plenty of water throughout the day.

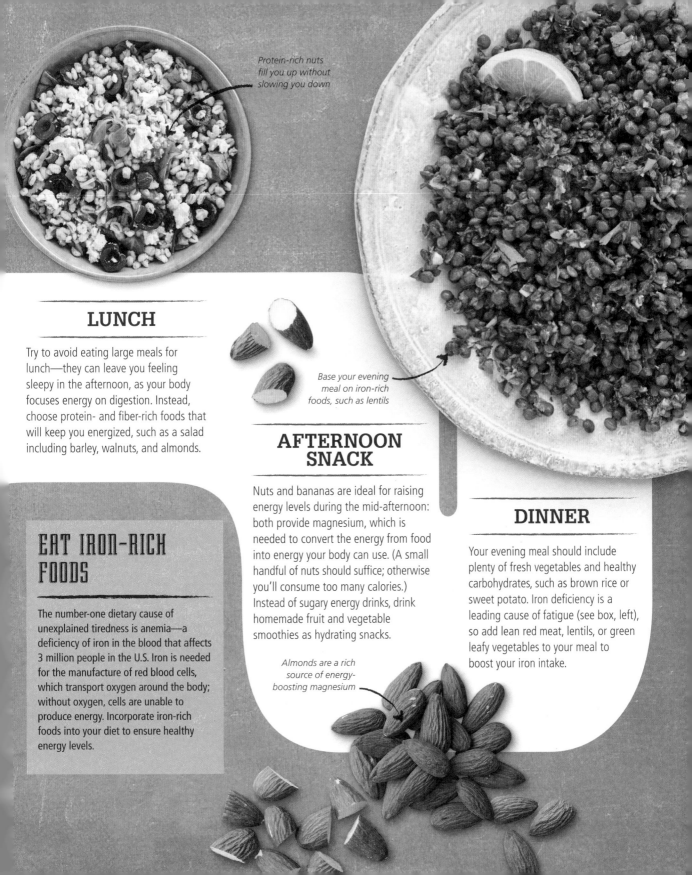

Protein-rich nuts fill you up without slowing you down

Base your evening meal on iron-rich foods, such as lentils

LUNCH

Try to avoid eating large meals for lunch—they can leave you feeling sleepy in the afternoon, as your body focuses energy on digestion. Instead, choose protein- and fiber-rich foods that will keep you energized, such as a salad including barley, walnuts, and almonds.

AFTERNOON SNACK

Nuts and bananas are ideal for raising energy levels during the mid-afternoon: both provide magnesium, which is needed to convert the energy from food into energy your body can use. (A small handful of nuts should suffice; otherwise you'll consume too many calories.) Instead of sugary energy drinks, drink homemade fruit and vegetable smoothies as hydrating snacks.

Almonds are a rich source of energy-boosting magnesium

EAT IRON-RICH FOODS

The number-one dietary cause of unexplained tiredness is anemia—a deficiency of iron in the blood that affects 3 million people in the U.S. Iron is needed for the manufacture of red blood cells, which transport oxygen around the body; without oxygen, cells are unable to produce energy. Incorporate iron-rich foods into your diet to ensure healthy energy levels.

DINNER

Your evening meal should include plenty of fresh vegetables and healthy carbohydrates, such as brown rice or sweet potato. Iron deficiency is a leading cause of fatigue (see box, left), so add lean red meat, lentils, or green leafy vegetables to your meal to boost your iron intake.

BAOBAB POWDER

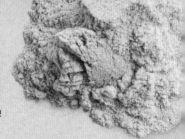

Baobab, derived from the fruit of Africa's "tree of life," is loaded with antioxidants, vitamin C, and fiber. It's good for your skin and gut, and helps protect against disease.

WHY EAT IT?

HIGH IN FIBER

Baobab powder is a good source of both soluble and insoluble fiber. Soluble fiber helps your body remove excess cholesterol from your blood, and also helps to slow down the release of sugar into the bloodstream, which prevents unhealthy spikes in energy. Insoluble fiber keeps your digestive system healthy, and helps reduce the risk of constipation, hemorrhoids, and diverticular disease.

DISEASE PREVENTION

Baobab is particularly rich in antioxidants—some reports suggest that baobab may contain more of them than any other fruit. Antioxidants help to neutralize free radicals, unstable molecules that can disrupt healthy cells and lead to heart disease, cancer, dementia, and Alzheimer's disease.

SKIN HEALTH

The vitamin C in baobab helps to keep your skin looking youthful. It helps to neutralize free radicals that accelerate wrinkling and other signs of aging, and also helps to form collagen, a protein that supports your skin.

WHAT'S IN IT?

1½ tablespoons of baobab powder is a good source of vitamin C, fiber, potassium, and magnesium. Baobab also contains vitamins B1 and B6, as well as calcium and iron.

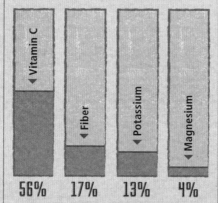

Vitamin C	Fiber	Potassium	Magnesium
56%	17%	13%	4%

Percentage of your daily reference intake

WHERE IS IT FROM?

Baobab is the fruit of an African tree. The fruit dries naturally on the plant, and after harvest it is ground to a powder.

Large green pods contain a powdery white pulp

HOW TO EAT IT

1 **SPARKLING DRINK**
Baobab powder has a bright, citrusy flavor. Blend it with a little water to make a paste, then top with sparkling water for a refreshing drink.

2 **IN OATMEAL**
Stir a little baobab powder into your morning oatmeal to give it a fruity boost. Serve with sliced bananas and slivers of raw almonds.

3 **BAOBAB SMOOTHIE**
Its sherbertlike taste makes baobab a great addition to a smoothie. Try it with tropical ingredients, such as mango, papaya, and coconut water.

MAXIMIZE THE BENEFITS

USE RAW POWDER
Preserve baobab's vitamin content by using it in cold dishes or adding it at the end of cooking. It can be used in baking, as it retains fiber and minerals when heated, but heating will reduce levels of vitamin C.

LUCUMA POWDER

The powdered pulp of the lucuma fruit is rich in antioxidant beta-carotene. Sweet and butterscotch-like, it makes a good substitute for sugar.

WHY EAT IT?

SKIN HEALTH
Beta-carotene in lucuma helps keep your skin bright and healthy. Research carried out at Rutgers University suggests that lucuma may have anti-aging properties and help promote wound healing.

HORMONE BALANCE
Lucuma powder is naturally sweet but has a low GI. This means that, unlike sugar, it doesn't cause spikes in blood-sugar levels, so the body doesn't have to respond by producing as much insulin. It may also help curb sugar cravings and appetite.

DISEASE PREVENTION
The phytochemical beta-carotene, which is found in lucuma, is known to help reduce the risk of certain types of cancer. It may also help boost your immune system and have antibacterial properties.

WHAT'S IN IT?

3½oz (100g) of lucuma powder provides a useful source of vitaminS B1 and B2, as well as phosphorus and calcium. Lucuma also contains iron, zinc, and niacin.

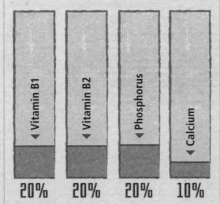

Vitamin B1	Vitamin B2	Phosphorus	Calcium
20%	20%	20%	10%

Percentage of your daily reference intake

WHERE IS IT FROM?

Cultivated 2,000 years ago by the Incas, lucuma is a fruit native to the Andean valleys. The fruit pulp is dried and ground to make powder.

Fruits contain vibrant orange flesh

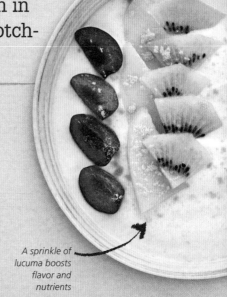

A sprinkle of lucuma boosts flavor and nutrients

Breakfast bowl ▲

HOW TO EAT IT

1 BREAKFAST BOWL
Sweeten a bowl of yogurt or oatmeal and fresh fruit with the caramel-like flavor of lucuma powder instead of honey or maple syrup.

2 HYDRATING DRINK
Sweeten water with lucuma powder in place of fruit juice. Add a spoonful of lucuma powder to filtered water, and stir or shake until dissolved.

3 IN CHIA PUDDING
Mix almond or coconut milk and chia seeds with 1 teaspoon of lucuma powder for a maplelike flavor. Leave the pudding to thicken overnight.

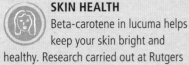

ACAI POWDER

Acai powder contains very high levels of disease-fighting antioxidants, as well as useful quantities of vitamin A, which supports your immune system.

WHY EAT IT?

HIGH IN ANTIOXIDANTS
Some studies suggest that acai contains more antioxidants than blueberries, specifically anthocyanins, phytochemicals that are known to be associated with a reduced risk of heart disease, stroke, and some types of cancer.

IMMUNE BOOST
Acai powder is a good source of vitamin A, which your body uses to keep your immune system functioning.

WHERE IS IT FROM?

Native to Central and South America, the acai palm commonly grows in the Amazon River estuary. Acai berries perish quickly once picked, so they are either dried and powdered or frozen for export.

Acai berries grow on large, branching stems

WHAT'S IN IT?

1 cup of acai powder provides a good source of vitamin A, potassium, calcium, and iron, as well as containing phytochemicals such as anthocyanins.

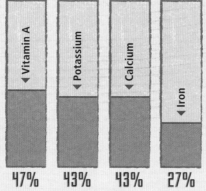

▼ Vitamin A	▼ Potassium	▼ Calcium	▼ Iron
47%	43%	43%	27%

Percentage of your daily reference intake

Acai energy balls ▶

HOW TO EAT IT

1 BREAKFAST
Acai has a sweet, tart taste that you can enjoy raw. Sprinkle the powder over granola or stir into yogurt or oatmeal.

2 BERRY SMOOTHIE
Add acai powder to a smoothie of blueberries, banana, and almond milk for an antioxidant-rich drink.

3 ACAI ENERGY BALLS
Cook fresh blueberries until softened, and mix in acai powder, rolled oats, pumpkin and sunflower seeds, and goji berries. Allow the mixture to cool before rolling into bite-sized balls. Firm up in the fridge before eating.

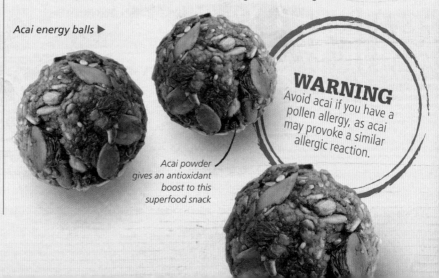

Acai powder gives an antioxidant boost to this superfood snack

WARNING
Avoid acai if you have a pollen allergy, as acai may provoke a similar allergic reaction.

NUTRITIONAL YEAST

Nutritional yeast is a type of fungus that provides an excellent source of many B vitamins, which help provide energy for your body and support blood health.

WHY EAT IT?

ENERGY BALANCE
Exceptionally high in several B vitamins, nutritional yeast helps your body access the energy in foods. A deficiency in B vitamins can lead to fatigue.

IMMUNE BOOST
Nutritional yeast contains a number of phytochemicals that may help strengthen your immune system.

BLOOD HEALTH
Nutritional yeast is usually fortified with vitamin B12, a vitamin often lacking in a vegan diet. Vitamin B12 is needed for the manufacture of red blood cells.

WHERE IS IT FROM?

Nutritional yeast, a type of fungus, is grown on sugar cane or molasses, before being processed into powder or flakes.

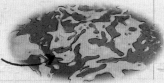

The yeast is washed and heat-treated to deactivate it

WHAT'S IN IT?

1 tablespoon of nutritional yeast provides an excellent source of vitamins B1, B6, and B12, as well as folate. It also contains vitamin B2, zinc, copper, and manganese.

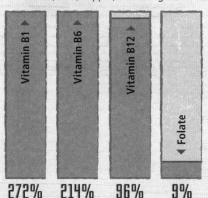

Vitamin B1	Vitamin B6	Vitamin B12	Folate
272%	214%	96%	9%

Percentage of your daily reference intake

Nutritional yeast comes as either powder or flakes

Nutritional yeast flakes ▲

HOW TO EAT IT

1 STIR-FRY SEASONING
Nutritional yeast has a deeply savory taste, and dissolves easily. Try sprinkling it on brown rice stir-fries for a hit of umami flavor.

2 ADD TO MASHED POTATOES
Adding nutritional yeast to mashed potatoes gives them a rich flavor without the need for adding cream or butter.

3 FLAVORED POPCORN
Nutritional yeast has a rich, cheesy taste that complements freshly popped corn. Add 1 tablespoon of coconut oil to the popcorn, sprinkle liberally with nutritional yeast flakes, and toss together well.

TIP
Not all brands of nutritional yeast are a good source of B12, so check the nutritional label and compare brands before you buy.

CACAO

Cacao is nutrient-rich when consumed raw. Phytochemicals found in cacao help keep your heart healthy and boost your mood, while manganese supports your blood, brain, and nerves.

WHY EAT IT?

HEART HEALTH
Cacao contains a group of phytochemicals called flavonoids, antioxidants that are linked with a reduced risk of heart disease. They are believed to work by helping to boost production of good HDL cholesterol and reduce blood pressure.

HIGH IN MANGANESE
The high levels of manganese in cacao support many of the chemical processes that occur in your body, including energy production. This vital mineral helps keep your blood, brain, and nerves healthy, and studies suggest that it may also help control blood sugar levels and prevent osteoporosis.

HORMONE BALANCE
The phytochemical phenylethylamine (PEA), which is found in cacao, boosts production of serotonin in the brain. Serotonin is known as the "feel-good" hormone, as it promotes feelings of happiness and well-being.

Flavonoids in cacao **reduce** the risk of **heart disease** by helping boost production of **good cholesterol**.

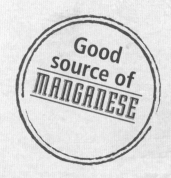

Good source of MANGANESE

WHAT'S IN IT?

½ cup of cacao nibs provide a good source of manganese, magnesium, iron, and potassium. Cacao nibs also contain calcium and zinc.

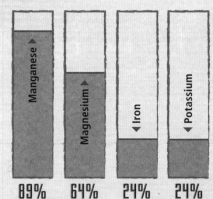

Manganese	Magnesium	Iron	Potassium
89%	64%	24%	24%

Percentage of your daily reference intake

Cacao nibs ▼

Cacao nibs are cracked, dehulled cacao beans

Cacao powder ▼

Raw cacao powder is made from unroasted, antioxidant-rich cacao beans

Cacao contains **high levels** of the vital mineral **manganese**, which is important for many of the **chemical processes** that occur in your body, including **energy production**.

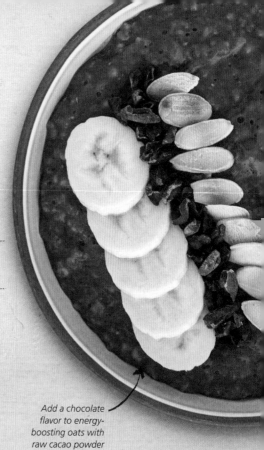

Add a chocolate flavor to energy-boosting oats with raw cacao powder

▲ Cacao oatmeal

WHERE IS IT FROM?

Cacao originates in Central America and the Amazon basin, and was transported all over the world by European colonialists. Cacao trees grow in humid, tropical conditions within the area 20 degrees north and south of the equator, but most of the world's production comes from small plantations in West Africa. Cacao trees take up to 5 years to mature and produce cacao pods. Pods are harvested for their flavorful beans, which are fermented, dried, and dehulled to form edible "nibs."

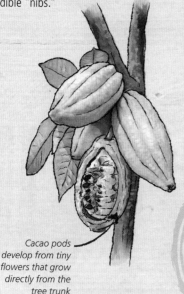

Cacao pods develop from tiny flowers that grow directly from the tree trunk

HOW TO EAT IT

1 CACAO OATMEAL

Cook rolled oats with almond milk and 3 teaspoons of raw cacao powder until softened to your liking. Sweeten with a little honey and top with cacao nibs, sliced banana, and toasted almonds for a nutritious breakfast.

2 IN ENERGY BARS

Add a handful or two of raw cacao nibs to raw energy bars (see pp48–49) for added nutty flavor, minerals, and heart-healthy phytochemicals.

3 IN BAKING

Use raw cacao powder in baking. Raw cacao products tend to have a more acidic, grassy flavor than their roasted counterparts, so sweeten your recipes with a little honey.

TIP

"Cacao" and "cocoa" refer to the same product, but "cacao" is often used on labels for raw products.

MAXIMIZE THE BENEFITS

CHOOSE RAW

Raw cacao products are made from unroasted cacao beans and contain higher levels of beneficial antioxidants than roasted beans.

EAT NATURAL

Cacao is a nutrient-rich natural product, but processing it into chocolate using high quantities of added fat and sugar negates many of its health benefits. Eat cacao in the form of powder or nibs to get maximum nutritional benefits.

SPIRULINA

Spirulina is a rich source of phytochemicals and energy-boosting B vitamins, as well as copper, which supports your bones and blood.

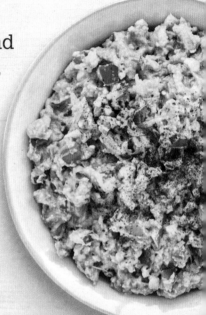

WHY EAT IT?

IMMUNE BOOST
Early studies suggest that three phytonutrients in spirulina—phycocyanin, polysaccharides, and sulfolipids—may greatly strengthen your immune system.

ENERGY BALANCE
Spirulina contains six B vitamins: thiamine, riboflavin, niacin, pantothenic acid, pyridoxine, and folate. These are involved in converting energy from food into energy the body can use. Some research suggests spirulina may improve energy levels in people with chronic fatigue syndrome and boost endurance for exercise.

Spirulina is most commonly sold as powder, but it is also available in flakes, capsules, and tablets

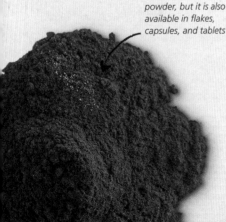

WHAT'S IN IT?

3½oz (100g) of spirulina powder is a good source of copper, vitamins B2 and B1, and iron. Spirulina also contains other B vitamins, as well as vitamins K and D.

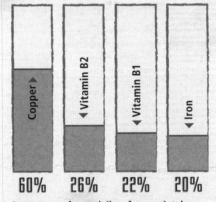

Copper ▲	▲ Vitamin B2	▲ Vitamin B1	▲ Iron
60%	**26%**	**22%**	**20%**

Percentage of your daily reference intake

WHERE IS IT FROM?

Spirulina is a type of algae that grows in fresh- and saltwater. It is dried before being processed.

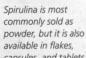

These algae are harvested from clean water

Spirulina guacamole ▲

HOW TO EAT IT

1 SPIRULINA GUACAMOLE
Combine 1–2 teaspoons of spirulina with four ripe, mashed avocados, a chopped tomato, finely diced red onion, a little garlic, and a handful of chopped cilantro.

2 GREEN RICE
The blue-green color of this algae is really outstanding. Add interest to pale dishes, such as a simple brown rice recipe, for a pop of color and added nutrients.

3 IN A SMOOTHIE
Spirulina powder has a strong taste and dark green color. A little goes a long way, so add it a little at a time to green smoothies, and taste as you go.

CHLORELLA

An excellent source of blood-healthy iron, chlorella may also help control blood sugar levels, protect against disease, and support digestive health.

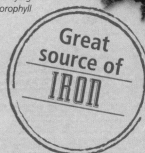

The green of chlorella powder is due to detoxifying chlorophyll

WHY EAT IT?

BLOOD HEALTH
According to some studies, chlorella may help people with diabetes control their blood sugar levels by affecting the genes that control insulin use in their body.

DISEASE PREVENTION
Some evidence suggests chlorella may help boost the immune system, protecting the body against infections. Chlorella may help reduce high blood pressure, which reduces the risk of heart disease. It may also help combat chronic conditions, including fibromyalgia and ulcerative colitis.

DIGESTIVE HEALTH
It has been shown that chlorella stimulates peristalsis—the muscular contractions that move waste material through the digestive tract. Chlorella is also believed to encourage the growth of healthy bacteria in the lower gut and to prevent toxic material in your digestive tract from being reabsorbed into the body.

WHAT'S IN IT?

2 teaspoons of chlorella powder is rich in iron and zinc, as well as vitamins B2 and B6. It also contains vitamins A, B1, B12, C, E, and K1, as well as niacin and folate.

Iron	Zinc	Vitamin B2	Vitamin B6
93%	71%	30%	10%

Percentage of your daily reference intake

WHERE IS IT FROM?

Chlorella grows in freshwater lakes in Japan and Taiwan. After harvesting, it is dried to paste and crushed to a powder.

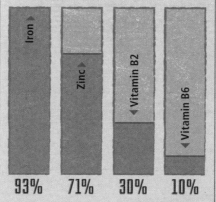

Chlorella is a type of single-cell algae

Great source of **IRON**

HOW TO EAT IT

1 CHLORELLA SMOOTHIE
Blend this health-giving powder, which has an intense, earthy flavor, with strong tastes, such as pineapple and mango, for a vividly colored morning smoothie.

2 ADD TO PESTO
If you want to hide rather than highlight the color and taste of these algae derivatives, blend them with brightly colored, strong-tasting dishes such as homemade pesto.

3 IN A SALAD DRESSING
Add ¼ teaspoon of chlorella powder to a salad dressing that includes puréed avocado, garlic, and lemon, and use to drizzle over raw vegetables or salads.

NUTRITION KNOW-HOW

To keep your body healthy, you need to consume particular quantities of nutrients each day. Your body's nutritional needs can usually be met by eating a varied diet based on nutritious whole foods, including plenty of superfoods. These pages detail recommended nutritional intakes for adults.

MACRONUTRIENTS

These nutrients are found in large quantities in food, and form the foundation of a healthy diet. Macronutrients provide your body with the tools it needs to function on a day-to-day basis. The quantity of each macronutrient that your body needs varies for each individual—here are guidelines for an average adult.

MACRONUTRIENTS	Daily reference intake for women	Daily reference intake for men
Energy	2000cals (8,400kJ)	2500cals (10,500kJ)
Carbohydrate - of which sugars	260g *no more than 50g added sugar*	330g *no more than 50g added sugar*
Fiber	30g	30g
Fat - of which saturated	*no more than 70g* *no more than 20g*	*no more than 90g* *no more than 30g*
Salt	*no more than 6g*	*no more than 6g*
Protein	50g	90g

MICRONUTRIENTS

Your body needs vitamins and minerals, or "micronutrients," as well as macronutrients in order to function. Men and women at different stages of life have different micronutrient needs—these charts show you the approximate quantities that you should aim to consume each day. Nutritional graphics in this book are based on suggested intakes for women aged 19–50.

VITAMINS	MEN 19–50	WOMEN 19–50	MEN 51–64	WOMEN 51–64	MEN 65–74	WOMEN 65–74	MEN 75+	WOMEN 75+
Vitamin A	700mcg	600mcg	700mcg	600mcg	700mcg	600mcg	700mcg	600mcg
Vitamin B1	1mg	0.8mg	0.9mg	0.8mg	0.9mg	0.8mg	0.9mg	0.8mg
Vitamin B2	1.3mg	1.1mg	1.3mg	1.1mg	1.3mg	1.1mg	1.3mg	1.1mg
Vitamin B3 (niacin)	17mg	13mg	16mg	12mg	16mg	12mg	16mg	12mg
Vitamin B5 (panthothenic acid)	*6mg*	*6mg*	*6mg*	*6mg*	*6mg*	*6mg*	*6mg*	*6mg*
Vitamin B6 (pyridoxine)	1.4mg	1.2mg	1.4mg	1.2mg	1.4mg	1.2mg	1.4mg	1.2mg
Vitamin B7 (biotin)	*50mcg*	*50mcg*	*50mcg*	*50mcg*	*50mcg*	*50mcg*	*50mcg*	*50mcg*
Vitamin B12	1.5mcg	1.5mcg	1.5mcg	1.5mcg	1.5mcg	1.5mcg	1.5mcg	1.5mcg
Folate	200mcg	200mcg	200mcg	200mcg	200mcg	200mcg	200mcg	200mcg
Vitamin C	40mg	40mg	40mg	40mg	40mg	40mg	40mg	40mg
Vitamin D	10mcg	10mcg	10mcg	10mcg	10mcg	10mcg	10mcg	10mcg
Vitamin E	*12mg*	*12mg*	*12mg*	*12mg*	*12mg*	*12mg*	*12mg*	*12mg*
Vitamin K	*75mcg*	*75mcg*	*75mcg*	*75mcg*	*75mcg*	*75mcg*	*75mcg*	*75mcg*

MINERALS	MEN 19–50	WOMEN 19–50	MEN 51–64	WOMEN 51–64	MEN 65–74	WOMEN 65–74	MEN 75+	WOMEN 75+
Calcium	700mcg	700mg	700mcg	700mg	700mcg	700mg	700mcg	700mg
Chromium	*40mcg*	*40mcg*	*40mcg*	*40mcg*	*40mcg*	*40mcg*	*40mcg*	*40mcg*
Copper	1.2mg	1.2mg	1.2mg	1.2mg	1.2mg	1.2mg	1.2mg	1.2mg
Magnesium	300mg	270mg	300mg	270mg	300mg	270mg	300mg	270mg
Phosphorus	550mg	550mg	550mg	550mg	550mg	550mg	550mg	550mg
Potassium	3500mg	3500mg	3500mg	3500mg	3500mg	3500mg	3500mg	3500mg
Iron	1.2mg	1.2mg	1.2mg	1.2mg	1.2mg	1.2mg	1.2mg	1.2mg
Zinc	9.5mg	7mg	9.5mg	7mg	9.5mg	7mg	9.5mg	7mg
Manganese	*2mg*	*2mg*	*2mg*	*2mg*	*2mg*	*2mg*	*2mg*	*2mg*
Iodine	140mcg	140mcg	140mcg	140mcg	140mcg	140mcg	140mcg	140mcg
Selenium	75mcg	60mcg	75mcg	60mcg	75mcg	60mcg	75mcg	60mcg

Intakes are based on UK guidelines, where available. Quantities in *italics* are based on EU guidelines.

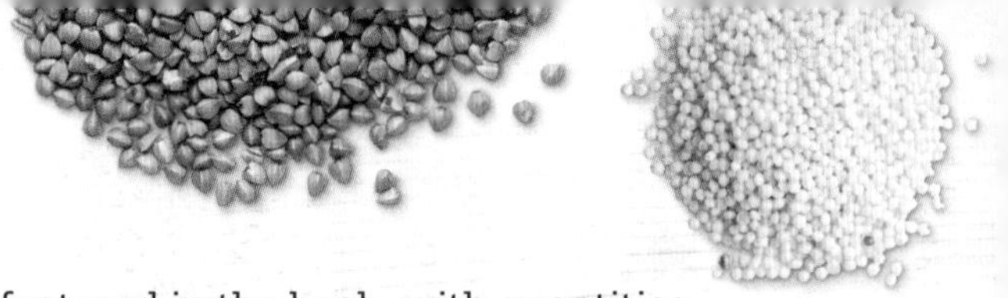

SUPERFOOD NUTRITION

These pages detail the key nutrients in each superfood featured in the book, with quantities in micrograms (mcg), milligrams (mg), or grams (g). Information is either given per 3½oz (100g) or, where appropriate, per serving. Key nutrients are those that are present in the superfood in particularly large quantities, or that are rare and found only in a few foods.

GRAINS

Superfood	Quantity or serving size	Key nutrients
Oats	1⅛oz / 40g (½ cup)	Beta-glucan 1.4g; vitamin B1 0.43mg; magnesium 46mg; zinc 0.92mg
Wheat germ	½oz / 15g (2 tbsp)	Manganese 2.02mg; vitamin B6 0.39mg; vitamin B1 0.25mg; vitamin E 2.43mg
Teff	7oz / 200g (¾ cup)	Vitamin B1 0.46mg; iron 5.7mg; fiber 7g; potassium 270mg
Barley	6¼oz / 180g (1 cup)	Selenium 69mcg; vitamin B1 1.2mg; beta-glucan 2.5g; magnesium 245mg
Brown rice	6¼oz / 180g (1 cup)	Manganese 1.66mg; selenium 18mcg; phosphorus 225mg; magnesium 86mg
Quinoa	6¼oz / 180g (1 cup)	Manganese 1.2mg; folate 78mcg; magnesium 118mg; iron 2.8mg
Amaranth	9oz / 250g (1 cup)	Manganese 2.1mg; phosphorus 364mg; magnesium 160mg; iron 5.2mg
Buckwheat	6¼oz / 180g (1 cup)	Copper 1.9mg; manganese 2.2mg; magnesium 392mg; fiber 17g

NUTS AND SEEDS

Superfood	Quantity or serving size	Key nutrients
Almonds	1oz / 28g (2 tbsp)	Vitamin E 6.7mg; biotin 19.8mcg; magnesium 76mg; calcium 67mg
Pistachios	1oz / 28g (¼ cup)	Copper 0.4mg; vitamin B6 0.4mg; potassium 300mg; protein 6g
Cashews	1oz / 28g (¼ cup)	Copper 0.59mg; manganese 0.48mg; phosphorus 157mg; magnesium 76mg
Pine nuts	1oz / 28g (¼ cup)	Manganese 2.5mg; copper 0.4mg; vitamin E 2.6mg; vitamin K 15mcg
Walnuts	1oz / 28g (¼ cup)	Manganese 1mg; copper 0.4mg; magnesium 44mg; fiber 2g
Peanuts	1oz / 28g (¼ cup)	Copper 0.29mg; vitamin B1 0.32mg; niacin 3.86mg; vitamin E 2.83mg
Brazil nuts	1oz / 28g (¼ cup)	Selenium 71mcg; copper 0.49mg; magnesium 115mg; vitamin E 2mg
Pumpkin seeds	1oz / 28g (½ cup)	Zinc 2.9mg; magnesium 76mg; iron 2.8mg; protein 8g
Sunflower seeds	1oz / 28g (¼ cup)	Vitamin E 10.6mg; vitamin B1 0.45mg; folate 64mcg; magnesium 109mg
Chia seeds	1oz / 28g (3 tbsp)	Manganese 0.6mg; magnesium 84mg; fiber 8.5g; phosphorus 265mg
Flaxseeds	1oz / 28g (3 tbsp)	Magnesium 110mg; manganese 0.7mg; vitamin B1 0.5mg; fiber 7.5mg
Sesame seeds	1oz / 28g (1 tbsp)	Copper 0.41mg; phosphorus 202mg; calcium 188mg; manganese 0.22mg
Alfalfa seeds	1oz / 28g (¼ cup sprouted)	Vitamin K 8.5mcg; folate 10mcg; vitamin C 3mg; magnesium 7.5mg

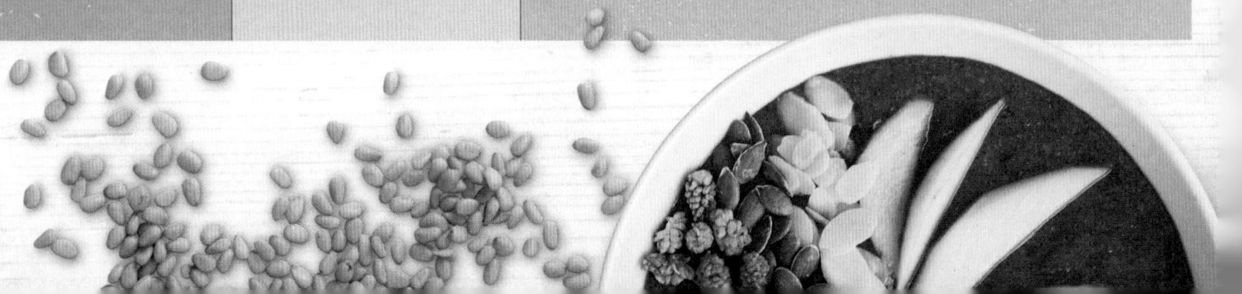

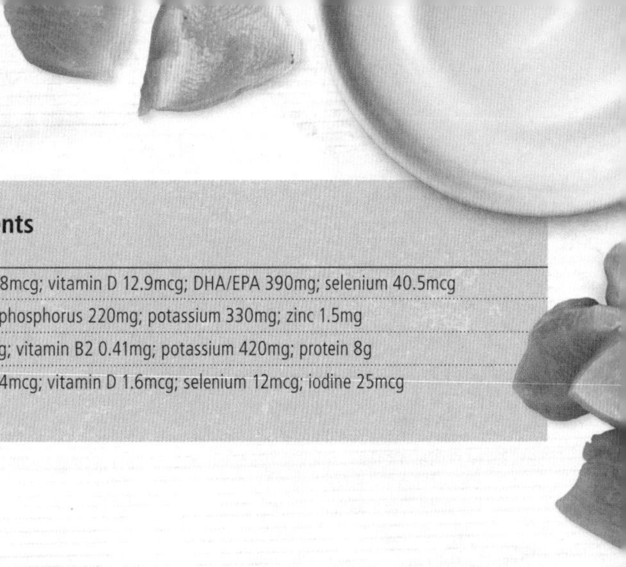

FISH, MEAT, DAIRY, AND EGGS

Superfood	Quantity or serving size	Key nutrients
Salmon	5½oz / 150g	Vitamin B12 9.8mcg; vitamin D 12.9mcg; DHA/EPA 390mg; selenium 40.5mcg
Chicken	3½oz / 100g	Niacin 9.2mg; phosphorus 220mg; potassium 330mg; zinc 1.5mg
Yogurt	5½oz / 150g (⅔ cup)	Calcium 300mg; vitamin B2 0.41mg; potassium 420mg; protein 8g
Eggs	2oz / 60g (1 large egg)	Vitamin B12 1.4mcg; vitamin D 1.6mcg; selenium 12mcg; iodine 25mcg

VEGETABLES

Superfood	Quantity or serving size	Key nutrients
Carrots	3½oz / 100g (¾ cup)	Vitamin A 1961mcg; vitamin K 13mcg; vitamin B1 0.13mg; potassium 178mg
Sweet potato	6¼oz / 180g (1 large sweet potato)	Vitamin A 1539mcg; vitamin C 41mg; manganese 0.9mg; potassium 846mg
Beets	3½oz / 100g (¾ cup)	Folate 150mcg; manganese 0.7mg; potassium 380mg; iron 1mg
Butternut squash	3½oz / 100g (½ cup cubed)	Vitamin A 545mcg; vitamin C 15mg; potassium 280mg; folate 19mcg
Fennel	3½oz / 100g (1 cup)	Potassium 876mg; folate 84mcg; vitamin C 12mg; fiber 3g
Onions	3½oz / 100g (¾ cup)	Folate 11mcg; vitamin B1 0.11mg; vitamin B6 0.1mg; potassium 138mg
Garlic	3½oz / 100g (¾ cup)	Potassium 620mg; phosphorus 170mg; vitamin C 17mg; manganese 0.5mg
Watercress	3½oz / 100g	Vitamin K 315mcg; vitamin C 62mg; vitamin A 420mcg; folate 45mcg
Spinach	3½oz / 100g	Folate 161mcg; vitamin C 29mg; potassium 682mg; vitamin A 260mcg
Kale	3½oz / 100g (1 cup)	Vitamin K 93mcg; vitamin C 110mg; vitamin A 525mcg; folate 120mcg
Cabbage	3½oz / 100g (1 cup)	Vitamin K 300mcg; vitamin C 96mg; folate 129mcg; potassium 513mg
Broccoli	3½oz / 100g (1 cup)	Vitamin K 127mcg; vitamin C 60mg; folate 72mcg; vitamin B1 0.29mg
Cauliflower	3½oz / 100g (¾ cup)	Vitamin K 28.5mcg; vitamin C 30mg; folate 48mcg; potassium 215mg
Shiitake mushrooms	3½oz / 100g (1 cup)	Copper 0.9mg; selenium 24.8mcg; vitamin B2 0.2mg; vitamin B6 0.2mg
Asparagus	3½oz / 100g (5 fat spears)	Folate 173mcg; vitamin K 51mcg; vitamin C 10mg; vitamin B1 0.12mg
Fava beans	3½oz / 100g (¾ cup)	Vitamin C 20mg; fiber 7g; niacin 3mg; folate 32mcg
Red kidney beans	3½oz / 100g (½ cup)	Manganese 0.5mg; folate 42mcg; potassium 420mg; iron 2.5mg
Peas	3½oz / 100g (¾ cup)	Vitamin B1 0.6mg; folate 50mcg; fiber 6g; iron 1.75mg
Lentils	3½oz / 100g (½ cup)	Selenium 16mcg; copper 0.13mg; manganese 0.2mg; iron 1.4mg
Red bell peppers	3½oz / 100g (1 cup)	Vitamin C 126mg; vitamin A 685mcg; copper 0.17mg; vitamin B6 0.23mg
Tomatoes	2½oz / 75g (1 medium tomato)	Vitamin C 16mg; folate 18mcg; potassium 167mg; vitamin K 4.5mcg
Avocados	3½oz / 100g (1 small avocado)	Vitamin E 3.2mg; vitamin B6 0.36mg; potassium 450mg; copper 0.19mg
Wakame	3½oz / 100g	Iodine 13,000mg; folate 196mcg; manganese 1.4mg; magnesium 107mg
Nori	¼oz / 10g	Vitamin B12 2.8mg; iodine 147mcg; vitamin A 238mcg; manganese 0.6mg

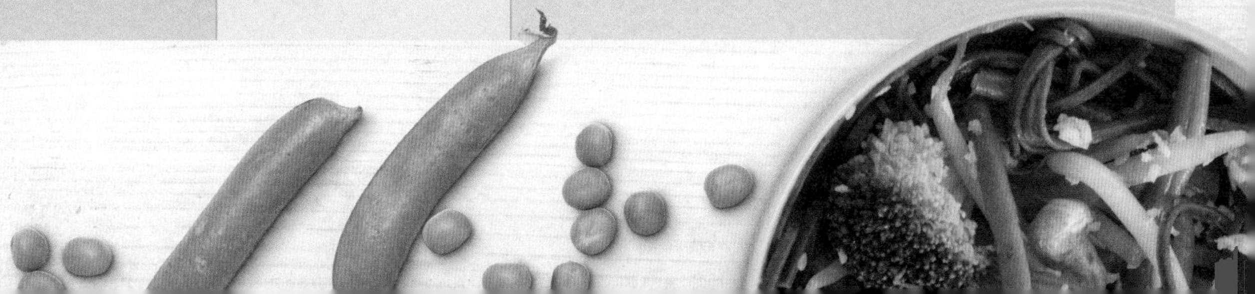

SUPERFOOD NUTRITION CONTINUED

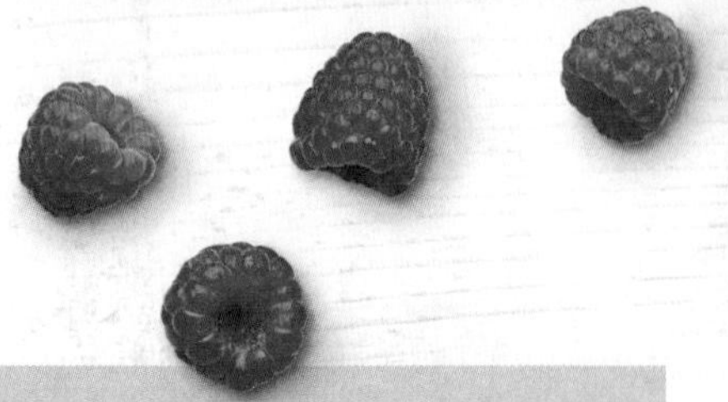

FRUIT

Superfood	Quantity or serving size	Key nutrients
Apple	5½oz / 150g (1 medium apple)	Vitamin C 9mg; vitamin K 8.4mcg; vitamin B6 0.11mg; potassium 150mg
Figs	3½oz / 100g (2 fresh figs)	Potassium 200mg; vitamin B6 0.08mg; calcium 38mg; zinc 0.3mg
Pomegranate	7oz / 200g (1 medium pomegranate)	Vitamin B6 0.6mg; vitamin C 26mg; fiber 9g; potassium 480mg
Plum	3½oz / 100g (½ cup)	Potassium 240mg; vitamin K 7.5mcg; copper 0.1mg; vitamin A 63mcg
Black currants	3½oz / 100g (¾ cup)	Vitamin C 200mg; potassium 370mg; manganese 0.3mg; vitamin B6 0.08mg
Cherries	3½oz / 100g (1 cup)	Vitamin C 11mg; potassium 210mg; copper 0.07mg; vitamin B6 0.05mg
Blueberries	3½oz / 100g (¾ cup)	Manganese 0.69mg; vitamin C 6mg; vitamin E 0.94mg; copper 0.06mg
Goji berries	1oz / 28g (2 tbsp)	Copper 0.6mg; vitamin B2 0.4mg; iron 2.5mg; potassium 235mg
Cranberries	3½oz / 100g (1 cup)	Manganese 0.4mg; vitamin C 13mg; fiber 4g; vitamin B6 0.07mg
Raspberries	3½oz / 100g (¾ cup)	Vitamin C 32mg; manganese 0.4mg; folate 33mcg; copper 0.1mg
Strawberries	3½oz / 100g (¾ cup)	Vitamin C 57mg; folate 61mcg; manganese 0.31mg; potassium 180mg
Banana	3½oz / 100g (1 medium banana)	Vitamin B6 0.31mg; manganese 0.36mg; potassium 330mg; vitamin B1 0.15mg
Pineapple	3½oz / 100g (½ cup)	Vitamin C 47.8mg; manganese 0.9mg; copper 0.11mg; potassium 160mg
Coconut	3½oz / 100g (1 cup shredded)	Manganese 1mg; copper 0.32mg; potassium 370mg; phosphorus 94mg
Oranges	5½oz / 150g (1 medium orange)	Vitamin C 56mg; vitamin B1 0.24mg; folate 34mcg; potassium 130mg
Lemons	3½oz / 100g (1 medium lemon)	Vitamin C 58mg; copper 0.26mg; vitamin B6 0.11mg; potassium 150mg
Guava	3½oz / 100g (½ cup, cubed)	Vitamin C 230mg; folate 49mcg; copper 0.2mg; potassium 417mg
Papaya	3½oz / 100g (¾ cup, cubed)	Vitamin C 60mg; folate 38mcg; vitamin A 135mcg; potassium 200mg
Mango	5½oz / 150g (1 medium mango)	Vitamin C 55mg; vitamin A 174mcg; vitamin B6 0.19mg; potassium 270mg
Kiwi	2oz / 60g (1 medium kiwi)	Vitamin C 74mg; vitamin K 24mch; folate 21mcg; potassium 174mg

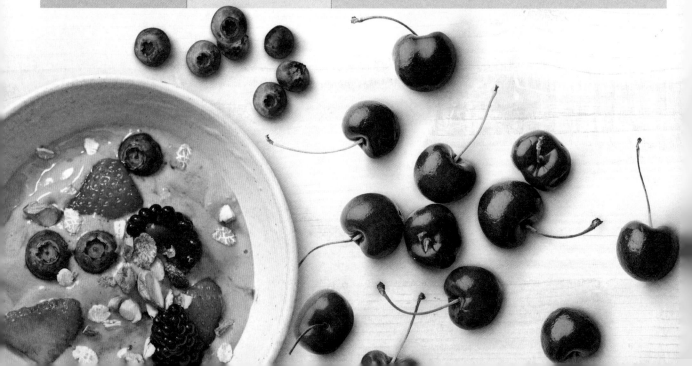

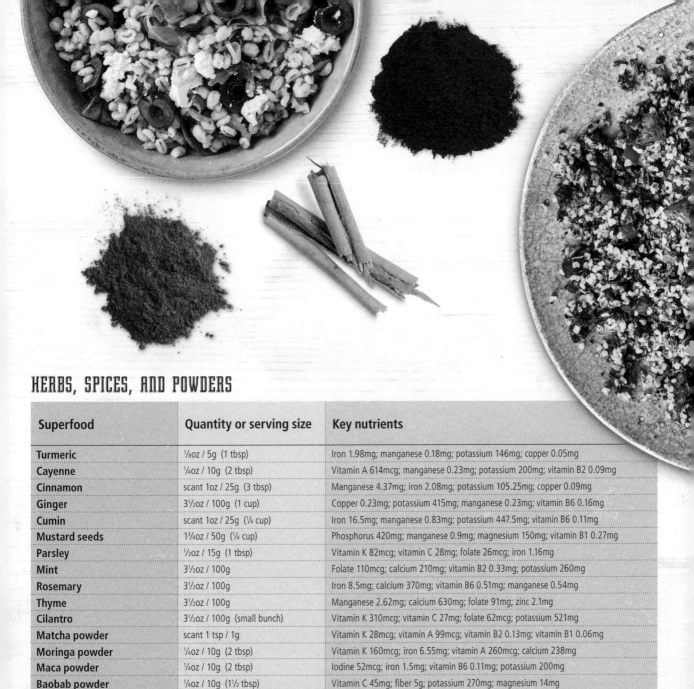

HERBS, SPICES, AND POWDERS

Superfood	Quantity or serving size	Key nutrients
Turmeric	1/8oz / 5g (1 tbsp)	Iron 1.98mg; manganese 0.18mg; potassium 146mg; copper 0.05mg
Cayenne	1/4oz / 10g (2 tbsp)	Vitamin A 614mcg; manganese 0.23mg; potassium 200mg; vitamin B2 0.09mg
Cinnamon	scant 1oz / 25g (3 tbsp)	Manganese 4.37mg; iron 2.08mg; potassium 105.25mg; copper 0.09mg
Ginger	3 1/2oz / 100g (1 cup)	Copper 0.23mg; potassium 415mg; manganese 0.23mg; vitamin B6 0.16mg
Cumin	scant 1oz / 25g (1/4 cup)	Iron 16.5mg; manganese 0.83mg; potassium 447.5mg; vitamin B6 0.11mg
Mustard seeds	1 3/4oz / 50g (1/4 cup)	Phosphorus 420mg; manganese 0.9mg; magnesium 150mg; vitamin B1 0.27mg
Parsley	1/2oz / 15g (1 tbsp)	Vitamin K 82mcg; vitamin C 28mg; folate 26mcg; iron 1.16mg
Mint	3 1/2oz / 100g	Folate 110mcg; calcium 210mg; vitamin B2 0.33mg; potassium 260mg
Rosemary	3 1/2oz / 100g	Iron 8.5mg; calcium 370mg; vitamin B6 0.51mg; manganese 0.54mg
Thyme	3 1/2oz / 100g	Manganese 2.62mg; calcium 630mg; folate 91mg; zinc 2.1mg
Cilantro	3 1/2oz / 100g (small bunch)	Vitamin K 310mcg; vitamin C 27mg; folate 62mcg; potassium 521mg
Matcha powder	scant 1 tsp / 1g	Vitamin K 28mcg; vitamin A 99mcg; vitamin B2 0.13mg; vitamin B1 0.06mg
Moringa powder	1/4oz / 10g (2 tbsp)	Vitamin K 160mcg; iron 6.55mg; vitamin A 260mcg; calcium 238mg
Maca powder	1/4oz / 10g (2 tbsp)	Iodine 52mcg; iron 1.5mg; vitamin B6 0.11mg; potassium 200mg
Baobab powder	1/4oz / 10g (1 1/2 tbsp)	Vitamin C 45mg; fiber 5g; potassium 270mg; magnesium 14mg
Lucuma powder	3 1/2oz / 100g	Vitamin B1 0.2mg; phosphorus 180mg; vitamin B2 0.3mg; calcium 90mg
Acai powder	3 1/2oz / 100g (1 cup)	Vitamin A 374mcg; potassium 860mg; calcium 347mg; iron 3.8mg
Nutritional yeast	1/8oz / 5g (1 tbsp)	Vitamin B1 3mg; vitamin B6 3mg; vitamin B12 2.4mg; folate 18mcg
Cacao nibs	3 1/2oz / 100g (1/2 cup)	Manganese 1.78mg; magnesium 240mg; iron 3.4mg; potassium 490mg
Spirulina	3 1/2oz (100g)	Copper 0.6mg; vitamin B2 0.37mg; vitamin B1 0.24mg; iron 2.8mg
Chlorella	1/4oz / 10g (2 tsp)	Iron 13mg; zinc 7.1mg; vitamin B2 0.43mg; vitamin B6 0.14mg

GLOSSARY

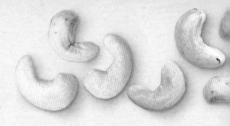

Anemia
A deficiency of red blood cells or hemoglobin usually related to a lack of iron or B vitamins.

Antioxidants
Chemicals found in fruit and vegetables that help counteract the damaging effects of free radicals on cells and tissues in your body.

Beta-glucan
A particularly effective form of soluble fiber, beta-glucan dissolves into a gel in your digestive tract and absorbs excess cholesterol.

Cholesterol
A waxy substance in your blood that forms part of cell walls, needed for your brain and nervous system. Excess cholesterol is deposited in the arteries, increasing the risk of heart disease and stroke.

Free radicals
Highly reactive molecules that are believed to be involved in the development of heart disease and some cancers, as well as increasing the risk of premature aging.

Fructooligosaccharides
A form of soluble fiber that encourages the growth of good bacteria in your gut.

Glycemic index (GI)
A measure of the rate at which carbohydrates are digested and converted into sugar, producing an increase in blood-sugar levels.

Hemoglobin
A protein in red blood cells that transports oxygen around your body.

HDL
High-density lipoproteins, or HDL, carry cholesterol away from tissues, helping to reduce the risk of heart disease. Also known as good cholesterol.

Insoluble fiber
A form of fiber that speeds the passage of waste material through your gut.

LDL
Low-density lipoproteins, or LDL, transport cholesterol to tissues and organs, and are linked with an increased risk of heart disease. Also known as bad cholesterol.

Macronutrients
Nutrients such as protein, carbohydrates, and fat that your body needs in large quantities. *See p212.*

Metabolism
A collective term for the chemical processes that occur in your body, including the conversion of energy from foods into energy your body can use.

Micronutrients
Vitamins and minerals that your body needs in small quantities. *See p213.*

Neural tube defects
Conditions affecting the health of a baby during the first month of pregnancy, including spina bifida.

Omega-3 fatty acids
A form of unsaturated fat that helps lower high blood pressure, protect against heart disease, and keep your brain healthy.

Oxidation
Damage caused to cells and tissues caused by free radicals. Oxidation can be neutralized by antioxidants.

Phytochemicals
Naturally occurring chemicals found in foods of plant origin. *See p16.*

Prebiotics
Forms of natural fiber that nourish gut-friendly bacteria.

Probiotics
Good bacteria that help keep your digestive system healthy.

Reference intakes
Based on official guidelines, reference intakes (RIs) provide a rough guide to how much of each nutrient you should aim to consume each day. RIs for each individual vary depending on age and gender.

Resistant starch
A form of starch that speeds the passage of waste material through your digestive system and encourages the growth of good bacteria in your gut.

Sarcopenia
Loss of muscle mass that is common in older people and can increase the risk of falls.

Saturated fat
A type of fat found in animal products, coconut oil, and palm oil that increases levels of bad cholesterol and the risk of heart disease.

Soluble fiber
Fiber that breaks down in the digestive tract, helping to reduce high cholesterol levels and slow the release of sugar into your blood stream.

Unsaturated fats
Healthy fats found in avocados, nuts, plant oils, and oily fish that help to lower high cholesterol levels and keep your heart and brain healthy.

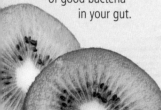

INDEX

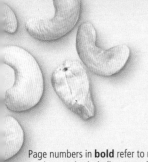
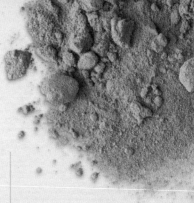

Page numbers in **bold** refer to main entries, entries in *italics* are recipes.

CONTINUED ▶

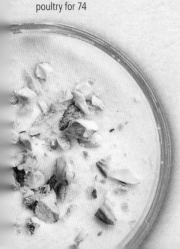
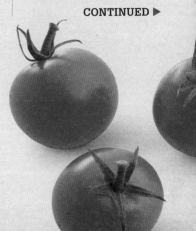

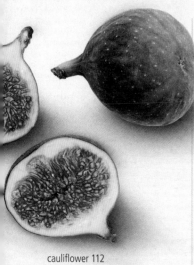

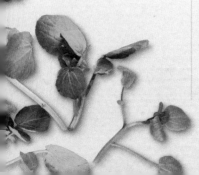

CONTINUED ▶

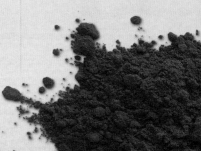

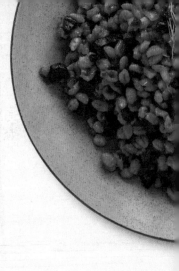

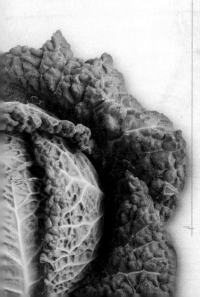

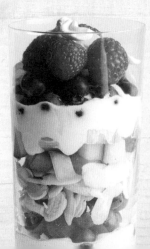

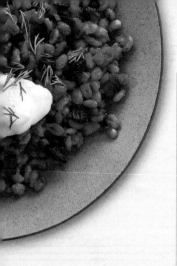
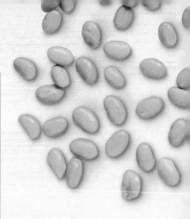

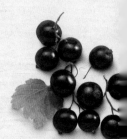

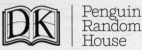
Penguin
Random
House

Editor
Alice Kewellhampton

Senior Designer
Kathryn Wilding

Designers
Mandy Earey and Dawn Terrey

Pre-Production Producers
Catherine Williams and Tony Phipps

Producer
Ché Creasey

Jackets Team
Libby Brown and Nicola Powling

Creative Technical Support
Sonia Charbonnier and Tom Morse

Managing Art Editor
Marianne Markham

Managing Editor
Dawn Henderson

Art Director
Maxine Pedliham

Publishing Director
Mary-Clare Jerram

US Managing Editor
Kayla Dugger

US Publisher
Mike Sanders

Botanical illustrations Peter Bull
Photography William Reavell

First American Edition, 2017
Published in the United States by DK Publishing
345 Hudson Street, New York, New York 10014

Copyright © 2017 Dorling Kindersley Limited
A Penguin Random House Company
2 4 6 8 10 9 7 5 3 1
001—294123—Jan/2017

Copyright © 2017 Dorling Kindersley Limited

All rights reserved.
Without limiting the rights under the copyright reserved
above, no part of this publication may be reproduced, stored
in or introduced into a retrieval system, or transmitted, in any
form, or by any means (electronic, mechanical, photocopying,
recording, or otherwise), without the prior written
permission of the copyright owner.
Published in Great Britain by Dorling Kindersley Limited.

A catalog record for this book is available
from the Library of Congress.
ISBN 978-1-4654-5629-8

DK books are available at special discounts when purchased
in bulk for sales promotions, premiums, fund-raising, or
educational use. For details, contact: DK Publishing Special
Markets, 345 Hudson Street, New York, New York 10014
SpecialSales@dk.com

Printed and bound in China

All images © Dorling Kindersley Limited
For further information see: www.dkimages.com

A WORLD OF IDEAS:
SEE ALL THERE IS TO KNOW
www.dk.com

ABOUT THE AUTHORS

Fiona Hunter is a food writer and nutritionist of over 30 years' experience. With a degree in nutrition and a postgraduate diploma in dietetics, she began her career as a dietician in the NHS before going on to write for magazines including *Good Housekeeping*, *Health and Fitness*, and *BBC Good Food*, as well as making many appearances on television and radio. She is the coauthor of several books, including *101 Fantastic GI Recipes*, *The Natural Menopause Cookbook*, and DK's *The Diabetes Cooking Book*.

Caroline Bretherton has worked in the food industry on both sides of the Atlantic for over 20 years. Her enthusiasm and skills led her to start her own catering company, and later a café, before going on to work consistently in television and the print media. She is the author of five cookbooks, including DK's *The Allotment Cookbook Through the Year* and *Family Kitchen Cookbook*. She lives in North Carolina with her family, from where she continues to write about all things food-related.

ACKNOWLEDGMENTS

Fiona Hunter would like to thank:
My Mum, who taught me how to cook, but more importantly to understand the importance of healthy eating—sadly she's not here to see the publication of this book, but I know she would have been proud. Big thanks also to my long-suffering husband for everything you do for me. Finally, thank you to Alice Kewellhampton from DK for her patience and support.

Caroline Bretherton would like to thank:
Everyone at DK for their professionalism and support, my family for their unwaiving ability to eat everything I put in front of them, and Laura Lascola for her enthusiasm for—and boundless knowledge of—all things superfoody.

DK would like to thank:
Rajdeep Singh for retouching images; Sunil Sharma for image management; Tia Sarkar, Arani Sinha, Martha Burley, Bob Saxton, and Alice Horne for editorial assistance; Charlotte Johnson and Alison Gardner for design assistance; Nicky Collings for photography art direction; Jane Lawrie and Penny Stephens for food styling; Rob Merrett for prop styling; Julian Shaw for checking botanical illustrations; Corinne Masciocchi for proofreading; and Marie Lorimer for indexing.

DISCLAIMER
Every effort has been made to ensure that the information in this book is accurate. However, the publisher is not responsible for your specific health or allergy needs that may require medical supervision, nor for any adverse reactions to the recipes contained in this book. Neither the authors nor the publisher will be liable for any loss or damage allegedly arising from any information or suggestion in this book.